True
Medical
Detective Stories

Other Books
by Clifton K. Meador, M.D.

A_Little Book of Doctors' Rules, Hanley & Belfus, 1992

With R. H. Lanius, *A Little Book of Nurses' Rules,* Hanley & Belfis, 1993

With W. Wadlington, *Pearls from a Pediatric Practice,* Hanley & Belfus, 1998

A Little Book of Doctors' Rules II, A Compilation, Hanley & Belfus, 1999

With C. M. Slovis and K. D. Wrenn, *A Little Book of Emergency Medicine Rules,* Hanley & Belfus, 2000

With W. Wadlington and M. Howington, *How to Raise Healthy and Happy Children,* iUniverse, 2001

Med School, Hillsboro Press, Providence Publishing Corporation, 2003

Symptoms of Unknown Origin, A Medical Odyssey, Vanderbilt University Press, 2005

Twentieth Century Men in Medicine: Personal Reflections, iUniverse, 2007

Puzzling Symptoms: How to Solve the Puzzle of Your Symptoms, Cable Publishing, 2008

Med School, Revised Edition. Cable Publishing, 2009

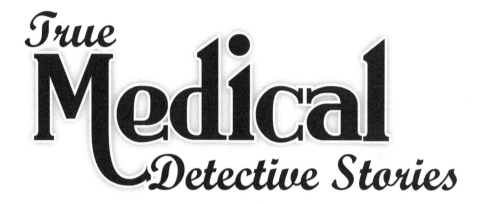

By

Clifton K. Meador, M.D.

Table of Contents

The most beautiful thing we can experience is the mysterious. It is the source of all true art and science.

— **ALBERT EINSTEIN**

Dedication

To Berton Rouché,
creator of Medical Detective Stories

Berton Rouché, author of *Eleven Blue Men* and *The Medical Detectives,* was a childhood hero of mine. My father gave me a copy of *Eleven Blue Men* when I was a teenager. I read the stories over and over, saying to my father that I wanted to be that kind of doctor when I grew up.

Rouché is best known for his medical detective stories, which were published frequently in the *New Yorker* beginning in 1944. In the fashion of Sherlock Holmes, he created the genre of the modern medical detective story. He became a regular contributor to the *New Yorker* with his "Annals of Medicine," publishing around two stories a year. He particularly liked medical mysteries that were solved by epidemiological methods.

Rouché read my earlier case report of Dr. Jim, which was published in the *New England Journal of Medicine,* and called me on the phone.[1] He asked if he could visit with me in Nashville to discuss the case in more detail. He spent a day taking notes and gathering the details of the case. He died before the case was published; however, the case was published later in a book with the title *The Man Who Grew Two Breasts.*[2] I was especially honored to have him write about one of my patients and then have him name the book after

---

1 C. V. DiRaimondo, A. Roach, and C. K. Meador, Gynecomastia, From Exposure of Vaginal Estrogen Cream, Letter, *New England Journal of Medicine* 1980; 302:1089–90.

2 B. Rouché, *The Man Who Grew Two Breasts* (New York: Truman Talley Books/Dutton, 1995).

Dr. Jim. (chapter 1 of this book is my version of the case of Dr. Jim's Breasts.)

I still puzzle over the irony and coincidence of meeting one of my childhood heroes and actually having him write a clinical case of mine. It was one of the high points of my medical career to meet and get to know Dr. Roueché, even though briefly. He died just a few months after I met him.

Roueché's influences on my practice of medicine and in the writing of this book are large. The medical detective stories and cases in this book are patterned after Roueché's methods of reporting. Mimicry, they say, is the highest form of flattery.

It gives me great pleasure to dedicate this book to the memory of Berton Roueché, the master of medical detective stories.

Acknowledgments

I want to thank many physician colleagues who shared or discussed their patients' clinical stories with me. Among these generous collleagues are Allen Kaiser, William Schaffner, William Hueston, Nortin Hadler, Anderson Spickard, Jr., William Stone, Marc Feldman, and Joseph Merrill. I especially want to thank Alan Graber, who gave suggestions that strengthened the telling of these stories.

Several friends offered constructive help, including Denette and Tom Blankenship, Virginia Fuqua-Meadows, JoniLea Stewart, and Bret Poe. I want to thank my daughter Ann Meador Shayne, an experienced author and editor, for her guidance in the process of making a book. I especially appreciate the efforts of the design team of CreateSpace. The book came to its final form through the fine editing efforts of Mary Neal Meador, wife of my son Clifton.

Many of the stories were first told in some of my other published books. The chapter notes at the end of the book give the primary references for those and other case reports.

Although the clinical features are all true, I have changed the names and identifying characteristics of all the patients and some of the physicians in order to protect their anonymity. Obviously, I have taken liberties with much of the dialogue. The chapter notes acknowledge those physicians who shared clinical stories with me.

I also want to thank my wife, Ann, for her support and editing skills.

Chapter One

Dr. Jim's Breasts

I had known Dr. Jim for many years. He practiced in a small town not too far from the city and had sent me a number of patients through the years. He was seventy-six years old and was complaining of breast enlargement when I saw him in 1977. The enlargement had started in the right breast. Because the enlargement was only on one side, it was thought he might have cancer of the breast. The right breast had been removed surgically before Dr. Jim asked me to see him. Cancer of the male breast is not a common lesion, but it does occur and can be quite malignant when it does.

Examination of the breast tissue did not show cancer, but it did show changes typical of "gynecomastia." Gynecomastia is the term to describe benign enlargement of the male breast. These changes are indicative of estrogen stimulation. The normally dormant male breast can be converted to a fully functioning "female breast" if the proper mix of female hormones is present in the bloodstream. The initial finding of one-sided breast enlargement was puzzling. Dr. Jim asked to see me when his remaining left breast had begun to enlarge.

I was not too confounded by the initial one-sided breast enlargement, because I had seen that before. There is sometimes a lag in the response of the breasts, and one will enlarge before the other even though the female hormone is available to both breasts. What did concern me was the appearance of gynecomastia at his age. It

1

usually meant the presence of a malignant tumor of the testicle or the adrenal gland.

At puberty, the normal male secretes both male and female hormones. Enlargement of the breasts in teenage boys is nearly universal if you examine carefully. This early influence of the female hormone is soon replaced by the dominant male hormone, which is secreted in increasing amounts. The effect of the female hormone is inhibited, and the breast enlargement is suppressed. At any time in later life, this same balance can be upset. If enough female hormone is present, breast enlargement will occur in the male at any age.

In the adult male, there are only two sources of female hormones, the testicles and the adrenal glands. Normally, both secrete small amounts of estrogens. Both, however, can develop tumors that are capable of secreting large amounts of estrogens. That was my first concern because these tumors are highly malignant—they grow and spread rapidly. There is a narrow window of time when surgical removal is still curative. In recent years, of course, effective hormone-based chemotherapy has become available for some of these tumors.

There is one other rare cause of estrogen secretion in the adult male: malignant tumors of various organs can curiously begin to make pituitarylike hormones that stimulate the adrenal or testicle to secrete estrogens. Lung cancer is one of these tumors that can produce this bizarre biochemical aberration.

With these ominous and serious possibilities in mind, I ordered all the tests that would identify the presence of estrogens or other hormones that can stimulate estrogen production. All the tests showed the low and normal levels of estrogens typical for a man his age. What a surprise! Knowing that false negative results can occur, I repeated the tests. Again the results came back within normal limits for a male.

My initial physical examination had been normal except for the easily felt gynecomastia of the remaining breast. I repeated the physical examination, this time spending extra time and attention on palpating his testicles for masses and pushing here and there in his abdomen, trying to feel his deep-seated adrenals. My examination was normal again. Had abdominal CAT scans been available at that time, I would have ordered one.

Not satisfied with these normal results and still quite concerned that there was a malignancy hidden away somewhere, I began to do x-rays and other procedures to find a tumor. My reasoning was that there are numerous compounds that can have an estrogen effect. The available tests only measured a small number of these compounds. Dr. Jim could be secreting a "hybrid" estrogen, if you will, and thus appear to have normal levels, because the tests I ordered were not "seeing" the novel hormone. It was a bit of fancy thinking, but I did not want to miss a malignancy that might still be surgically removable.

All of the imaging tests and procedures showed no tumors. I was in a blind-end alley. I had a colleague see him with me in consultation. He had no new thoughts but suggested repeating the tests once more, which we did, only to find the same normal results.

I then recalled a patient I had seen years before. He was a young boy, about six years old, who had developed gynecomastia at age five. Gynecomastia at that age is as ominous as it would be at Dr. Jim's age. The list of possibilities is just as full of cancers, if not more so. After an exhaustive but negative search for tumors, I began to look around for other causes. I had the mother bring in all the medicines in the house, thinking that the boy might be getting into her birth control pills or some estrogen-type compound. The only medicine was a vitamin the boy took on a routine basis.

A few months later, there was a report in a medical journal that a certain brand of vitamins had been contaminated with estrogens. Apparently, in the process of stamping the pills, the same press to make estrogen pills was used to press out the vitamin pills. Enough estrogen was carried over on the press to contaminate the vitamins. I immediately thought of the little boy who had me so puzzled and called his mother. Sure enough, the vitamins were the same brand. Stopping the vitamins led to a regression of the little boy's breasts back to normal within a few months. I was amazed at how such a minute dose of estrogen could produce such a profound physical effect.

When I thought of the little boy, I called Dr. Jim. I had taken a careful drug history when I first saw him and got no clue that he was taking anything that might have estrogen in it. I even had the nerve to ask him if he smoked marijuana, a frequent cause of gynecomastia in the drug subculture. After he laughed at my question, he asked me if I thought he was one of "those long-haired dope fiends." On the phone I asked if the wife took any estrogens, thinking somehow they might rub off on something he was using. I was fishing for any clue. He answered that she was not taking any.

I told him the story of the little boy and the contaminated vitamins. I asked him to think and see if he could come up with anything he was doing or taking that could stimulate the breasts to enlarge. By this time in my practice with patients who had puzzling symptoms, I had developed the habit of having them keep a diary of daily events. My intentions were to get them to search out for any hidden correlates in their lives that might affect their symptoms. I suggested this to Dr. Jim. He laughed and rejected the notion as silly.

I didn't see Dr. Jim for over a month. We had agreed to go along and see what happened. I was not at all satisfied with my inability to make a diagnosis for such an obvious and ominous abnormality. One day Dr. Jim showed up with his wife without an appointment. He was grinning and blurted out, "This was just too good to tell you over the phone. Gladys has made the diagnosis that you and I missed. Tell him, Gladys."

She went into great detail about their sex lives, how they had continued to "enjoy" each other frequently, sometimes several times a week. And then came the answer to the puzzle. For years she had used a vaginal cream for an atrophic vaginitis, a condition that can occur in older women due to the absence of estrogen. Not knowing what was in the cream, she began to check around after I asked Dr. Jim to keep a diary. Sure enough, it contained estrogen in a cream commonly prescribed to a lot of postmenopausal women for the same problem. She had started using the estrogen cream directly as a lubricant. Then she said, winking, "You don't suppose that has anything to do with Jim's breasts, do you?" And then she laughed out loud.

I just shook my head in disbelief. "We will certainly find out," I answered.

She had hit the diagnosis right on target. I knew the minute she told the story that she was right. Over several years he must have absorbed enough estrogen through the skin of his penis to produce breast enlargement but not enough to measure in the tests.

They stopped using the estrogen cream and within a few months the remaining breast returned to normal. The diagnosis was made. Gladys thought of it. I never would have.

Dr. Jim was one more example of the uniqueness of each patient. He illustrated vividly the principle that diseases can come from strange interactions between the infinite variety of stimuli from the world outside the body and the world of receptors inside the body. The trick in clinical medicine is to guide the patient to explore both worlds. Never in my wildest imagination would I have thought of asking Dr. Jim if his wife was using vaginal estrogen cream as a lubricant.

It is awesome to reflect on the number and variety of stimuli that exist in the world around us. Consider just for a moment the possible number of different substances we encounter in air and water. Add to that list the plants, clothing, air conditioning, heating, food additives, various dyes, soaps, lotions, and all the other compounds and chemicals, including vaginal estrogen creams. There is no way a physician or anyone can think of all the possibilities of toxic interactions that can occur. Add to that perplexity the notion that each of us is biochemically and physiologically unique. One man's biochemical hell is another's heaven. What will make some of us sick will have no influence on others.

It is blatantly obvious that only the individuals can begin to know the world around them. Certainly others can direct the patient to look at this or examine that, but in the long run people must figure out what is and is not affecting their health.

Again I relearned what I had been taught earlier. Sooner or later patients will tell you what is wrong if you listen carefully, especially if they are gently directed to look around themselves and wonder. Sometimes a physician has to listen for a long time, but it remains true that patients are their own best medical detectives.

Chapter Two

A Young Doctor and a Coal Miner's Wife

A young doctor, Dr. Bill Hueston, and his wife had just moved to the mountains of eastern Kentucky, near the border of West Virginia. The small town was nestled among the coal mines of the region. Nearly all of his patients would be coal miners or family members of a miner. Bill would practice family medicine. His wife, a veterinarian, hoped to build a small-animal practice.

Liz McWherther, the forty-seven-year-old wife of a miner, came to see the young doctor. Over several weeks, she had developed a curious set of complaints. Each morning she woke with a dry mouth and slurred speech. She also noted blurred vision and difficulty urinating. Within a couple of hours of waking, she was completely free of any symptoms. These symptoms had been occurring each morning and going away by afternoon.

Liz had had a series of tests done by the previous physician, but none of these tests were abnormal. The physical examination by Dr. Hueston was entirely normal. She denied drinking alcoholic beverages or using illicit drugs. Hueston had briefly considered some unusual response to marijuana or other drugs that were prevalent in the area. Liz had not been down in the mines, nor did her husband bring back anything unusual into the house.

The complex of symptoms suggested multiple sclerosis or some diffuse neurological disease. However, the rapid disappearance of the symptoms was puzzling. The most perplexing feature was the improvement as the day went on. Nearly all neurological diseases get worse as the day progresses. In most cases after a night's rest, the neurological circuits are improved, and patients are at their best on arising. Not so with Liz. She was at her worst on arising and rapidly improved within a few hours.

Dr. Hueston went through a long list of possible neurological conditions. None seemed to fit the findings or course of the symptoms. Hueston came to the conclusion that he needed a neurological consultation. The nearest neurologist was over fifty miles away, so he began filling out the request for consultation and other forms required by the miners' insurance.

Hueston was chatting as he wrote. "My wife and I are new to the area. You know she is a veterinarian. She's having a hard time dealing with the amount of skin disease in her patients. All of the cats and dogs are loaded with ticks and fleas. She didn't have that problem in her city practice."

Liz's attention became alert. "Yeah, I had that with my cat. But I fixed it."

"How'd you get it fixed?"

"I just dust her every week."

Hueston stopped writing and paused. "You dust her. What do you mean 'dust her'?"

"I just take my rose dust I use in my garden. Dust it on my cat. Then just rub it in."

Hueston asked, "Rose dust? What's that?"

"I don't know what all's in it. It kills the insects on the roses and it sure kills ticks and fleas on my cat. My cat is free of 'em."

Hueston, now in full alert, asked, "Where does the cat sleep?"

Liz smiled and answered, "Why, she sleeps right on my pillow with me."

Hueston said, "I want you to go home and wash your cat. Don't use the rose dust anymore, and don't let the cat in your room at night. Let's see what happens and maybe you won't have to go all the way to Lexington."

Liz came back a week later. Smiling widely, she told Dr. Hueston she had not had any more dry mouth, blurred vision, or slurred speech. Her urination was completely normal. The "disease" had gone away. She even brought a bag of the rose dust with her.

Dr. Hueston smiled back. He read the chemical contents on the rose dust bag and found what he suspected in the contents—organophosphates.

He went on to explain to Liz McWherther how organophosphates are nerve poisons. They cause some segments of the nervous system to fire continuously. The pupils constrict to pinpoint size. Salivation is inhibited. The urinary bladder does not function normally. If the exposure to organophosphates continues or the dose is large, death can occur.

Everyone wondered why the cat did not get sick. We will never know. Liz's problems were symptoms that she noted and described.

Cats don't talk.

A Paradoxical Suicide Attempt

Dr. Jesse Wilkins had just come on duty in the emergency room. He checked off with the outgoing medical resident, turned on CNN in the call room, and settled in for what he hoped would be a quiet evening. The bulk of the early evening crowd of patients had left, and no one was in the waiting room. A rare moment, Wilkins thought. He had no way of knowing how unusual his next patient would be.

Just as he was getting into Wolf Blitzer's discussion of the latest news from Iraq, the charge nurse called. "Better come see this one. He OD'd (overdosed) on something. Looks like shock to me."

Dr. Wilkins walked into the hallway just as they wheeled the patient's gurney into the exam room.

The patient, a young man, was pale and sweating profusely. His blood pressure was 80/40 and his pulse rate was 140. He kept blurting out, "Please. Help me. Took all my pills." He repeated this frequently in between his rapid breathing. "I don't want to die."

A neighbor who brought the patient to the ER said he had heard the patient call out from the hallway of the apartment building and then fall to the floor. The patient pointed to an empty bottle and told the neighbor that he had taken all of the remaining pills. He told the neighbor he made a mistake, that he did not want to die, and that he wished he had not taken the pills. He asked to be taken to the hospital.

Other than the low blood pressure and rapid pulse and breathing, the remainder of the physical exam was normal. The patient was conscious but lethargic with slurred speech. An intravenous line was inserted immediately and an infusion of saline was begun. Blood and urine samples were obtained for tests and for drug screening. The patient did not know the name of the drug he had taken.

The patient, Fred Mason, a twenty-six-year-old graduate student at the local college, had developed depression about one month earlier when his girlfriend dropped him. She told him that she could not tolerate his inability to make decisions. He became depressed and then saw an ad for a clinical trial of a new antidepressant. He decided to enroll to get the new drug. He had completed one month of the clinical trial and had just refilled the bottle one day before the suicide attempt. He had called his ex-girlfriend, and they got into an argument. Following the phone call, he immediately took all of the twenty-nine remaining pills, meaning to kill himself.

He explained that the pills he took were an experimental drug for depression. The label on the prescription bottle confirmed that the bottle contained capsules as part of a clinical trial of an antidepressant, but it did not indicate the name of the drug. In most clinical trials for new drugs, one half of a randomly selected group of patients gets the real drug to be tested. The other half of the group gets an inert pill—a placebo. This is usually a sugar pill made to look exactly like the real drug. Patients are not told if they are on the real drug or on the placebo; nor can patients tell from looking at the pill whether it is a real drug or inert. The clinical trial is to determine if the tested drug is more effective than a sugar pill. The code for who is getting the drug or who is getting the placebo is kept secret from both the trial doctors and the patients until the clinical trial is completed; hence, this kind of drug trial is called a double-blind trial.

Mason had a bout of depression when he was twenty-two years old and was treated with amitriptyline, an antidepressant. He stopped the medication because the drowsiness was intolerable and he had developed a numbness of his body. He thought the medication was too strong.

Mason's blood pressure rose with the intravenous saline but fell when the rate of infusion was slowed. Over four hours he received six liters of saline but remained lethargic, with a blood pressure of 100/62 and a pulse rate of 106. The drug screens of the urine were reported as negative, and the blood chemistries were within the normal range.

At this time, a physician from the clinical drug trials arrived in the emergency room. He had broken the code of the clinical trial as requested. He said that Mason had been assigned to the placebo group. The pills Mason had taken were, in fact, inert sugar pills. The patient had not received any active drug. When the patient was told this, he immediately expressed surprise and relief. Within a few minutes, his blood pressure rose to 126/80, and his pulse rate fell to 80. He became fully alert and was no longer drowsy.

The profound physiological changes and drop in blood pressure were all the effects of Mason's thinking and believing that he was taking a strong antidepressant. Mason's prior experience with negative side effects from an actual antidepressant may have reinforced his belief in the power of the pills he took for his attempted suicide. There is no stronger example of mind affecting body than this case—a nearly successful suicide from sugar pills.

After a few days in the psychiatric unit, Mason was started on the antidepressant sertraline, then discharged. He would be followed with psychotherapy as an outpatient.

This was the first reported case of attempted suicide with a placebo. Placebos are inert chemical agents. As they did with Mason, they can induce measurable chemical and physiological changes in some people. "Placebo" is Latin for "I will please." The so-called placebo effect can lead to desirable results, such as relief of pain, in susceptible people. When the effects are negative or undesirable, it is considered to be a "nocebo effect," from the Latin for "I will harm." Mr. Mason's harmful and near-death response to the inert substance is an example of the nocebo effect.

The positive response to placebos in clinical drug trials can be as high as 40 percent of the patients receiving them. In many cases it is difficult to distinguish placebo responders from those responding to an active drug. Both nocebo and placebo responses are under intensive studies in several research centers. The mechanisms for the induced responses are not yet clearly understood. What is quite clear is that certain people will react with measurable responses to chemically inert substances. This response can be negative or positive.

Mr. Mason, anticipating a fatal effect from the "drug" in his attempted suicide, clearly demonstrated a profound negative effect with lethargy, a rapid pulse, and a drop in blood pressure—all poorly responsive to intravenous saline.

There seems to be no limit to the effects that a firmly held belief can create in susceptible people. Mason believed he was taking a drug that was powerful enough to kill him, and his body began to respond as if he were actually dying. As soon as he was told the pills were placebos, his blood pressure, pulse rate, breathing, and level of consciousness immediately returned to normal.

Given the right situation and circumstances, the human mind seems infinitely plastic and malleable; it will believe almost anything. The body will respond to the dictates of the mind.

Chapter Four

A Curious Epidemic

On June 20, 1993, the sun had risen on a 15,000-acre idyllic retirement community located on the Cumberland Plateau in rural Tennessee. The emergency room staff at the small local hospital was about to change shifts. It was six thirty in the morning. Dr. Ernest Goodman was going over charts and signing his notes from the night before when the EMS ambulance pulled up to the entrance.

Two attendants called out to the nurse who was walking toward the ambulance, "High fever. Wife found him unconscious on the floor of their bathroom. Temp 104. Pulse 150. Not sure of BP."

They pulled the gurney out of the back of the ambulance and pushed the man through the glass doors of the ER. Dr. Goodman followed them down the hallway into the first treatment room. The nurse, her aide, and Goodman went into full action. They cut off the man's pajamas to see an obese, elderly man. His skin was pale blue but showing no rash. He was breathing fast, over forty breaths a minute. There was no response to pinching skin or to yelling verbal command. Tad Olsen was in a deep coma.

"Get me the ventilator. The man's in respiratory failure." The blood oxygen level was low but rapidly rose to normal with the ventilator and 100 percent oxygen.

After putting a tube into his airway and the ventilator in place, Dr. Goodman drew several tubes of blood before starting an intravenous line with normal saline. The tubes would be carried to the small lab for analysis and culture.

With the IV running, Goodman stepped back. "Where is the family or wife?" he asked.

The wife rushed into the exam room, having followed the ambulance in her car. She was breathing hard and shaking as she spoke. "Tad went to bed sick last night. Ached all over. Had a terrible headache. Told me he felt like the flu."

"When did all that start?" Dr. Goodman asked.

"Came on real sudden. He wasn't hungry for supper but came down sick right after we ate. Had trouble walking to bed. I checked him a couple of times during the night. Next thing I knew, I found him on the floor of the bathroom. Couldn't rouse him."

Dr. Goodman said, "Not many infections will take a grown man from health to near death so quickly. List is short. Spinal meningitis, or bloodstream infections like with strep—old fashioned blood poisoning, we used to call it. Flu and pneumonia, but they are a bit slower. And around here, the tick fevers, like Rocky Mountain spotted fever and a new one called erlichiosis."

A portable chest x-ray showed extensive whitening in both lung fields, indicating lungs full of fluid. He turned to the nurse and said, "Get the spinal tap tray."

As soon as Goodman performed the spinal tap and checked the spinal fluid under the microscope, he said, "Well, that rules out spinal meningitis. Will culture fluid anyhow." Goodman talked to himself as he went along.

Continuing to talk to himself, "Well. We've got a white-out chest x-ray, low oxygen. Normal spinal fluid. What's the blood count?" Goodman called out to the nurse, who also doubled as the lab tech.

"White count is 2300, very low," she answered from the small corner lab counter.

"Now add a low white count and shazam! We've got tick fever. No rash but not necessary. Get the tetracycline."

A few hours later, Olsen was making no urine and was clearly in kidney failure, necessitating hemodialysis over the next few days.

The next day, Olsen's neighbor, Jeff Smathers, came into the emergency room, barely able to walk from his wife's car. Smathers eventually had identical symptoms to Olsen—high fever, respiratory failure, kidney failure, and a low white count.

Both men required artificial ventilation and hemodialysis for support, and both men survived with no residual damage.

Special serological studies of their blood finally confirmed the diagnosis of erlichiosis several days later.

Between June 19 and June 25, in addition to Tad and Jeff, two other men would be admitted to the hospital with high fever, severe headaches, muscle aches, nausea, and abdominal pains. All four recalled a tick bite, but none of the men had any rash. Despite the absence of the expected rash, the local physicians, already alert to tick-borne disease, began tetracycline, the correct treatment for most such infections. By the end of summer, eleven cases of ehrlichiosis would be identified. There were no deaths. Ted and Jeff miraculously recovered, due to the expert care of their physicians.

The Center for Communicable Diseases and the Infectious Disease Division of Vanderbilt School of Medicine were called into consultation to study the epidemic of ehrlichiosis. This team of epidemiologists did an extensive study of the community, comparing it to a distant community in the same area. A random sample from the distant inhabitants was questioned and blood drawn for analysis.

The retirement and golfing community had been carved out of a wildlife-management area of over eighty thousand acres on the Cumberland Plateau in Tennessee. The three thousand year-round residents had access to four eighteen-hole golf courses. Both the homes and golf courses bordered on the large surrounding wildlife area. The Olsens and the Smathers enjoyed grilling out on their decks and watching deer and raccoons come into their yards. Often they saw foxes, opossums, and even an occasional skunk in the surrounding woods. Both couples believed they had moved from Michigan to a wildlife and golfing, Disney-like paradise; that is, until the serious illness struck a total of thirty residents that summer.

Analyses of the blood samples from the sick patients revealed evidence for infection with *Ehrlichia chaffeensis*, a rickettsial organism transmitted by the Lone Star tick (*Amblyomma americanum*). Rickettsia are a class of infectious agents carried by ticks and other vectors. Deer and raccoons carried the infected ticks. The first case of ehrlichiosis was described in 1987, only six years prior to this outbreak. Other well-known rickettsial diseases are Rocky Mountain spotted fever and Lyme disease. The usual annual incidence of ehrlichiosis in endemic areas is about three to five cases per one hundred thousand population. This epidemic, reported in the *New England Journal of Medicine* from the Cumberland Plateau, revealed a high attack rate of 330 per one hundred thousand population when retrospective and prospective cases were identified and included with the eleven active cases. The close proximity to the animals of the wildlife preserve seemed to be a factor in explaining the epidemic. The most puzzling unexplained feature in the epidemic was the predominance of males with the infection.

The epidemiologists found three factors increased the rate of infection: being male, not using insect repellent, and playing golf. Women, although they played as much golf as their husbands, somehow escaped the disease. What was it about male golfers that made them differ from female golfers?

Further analysis showed that the poorest golfers among the men were the ones most often infected. No par golfers were infected. The reason for this unusual gender difference became obvious: poor golfers slice more balls into the wooded roughs. Men, more so than women, went into the rough, thick with trees and bushes, to try to find and hit their balls. The women golfers ignored balls hit into the rough and simply dropped a new ball on the fairway. The roughs, filled with ticks carrying the *Ehrlichia* organism, led to infection in only the males, most of whom were poor golfers.

Neither Tad Olsen nor Jeff Smathers had ever broken a score of 100. Both men invariably went into the rough to find their balls. Their wives, Babs and Susan, ignored balls that went into the rough. It was too easy to drop a new ball in the fairway.

This case of gender difference was solved by the epidemiological detectives.

Chapter Five

A Strange Coincidence

Sometimes coincidences are so striking in their timing and occurrence that it is difficult not to assign divine intervention. Such was the case with an experience I had in the emergency room in late August 1961.

It was an unusually hot evening. As a second-year medical resident, I would be rotating in the emergency room for the next three months. Emergency rooms in the early 1960s bore little resemblance to those of the present day. We were still in the era of little or no health insurance and a strong belief by the public that medical care was a last resort. Hospitals were where people went to die. "An apple a day keeps the doctor away" was a popular saying. The scant use of emergency rooms was an example of those beliefs.

Duty in the ER was episodic, and I was in the middle of one of the frequent lulls in activity. I took the opportunity to scan the medical journals that had piled up in the on-call room. I had just finished reading the latest issue of the *New England Journal of Medicine,* published on August 10, just over a week past, when the nurse called me to come see a new patient.

The patient, a man, looked to be in his late forties. He was obviously a mechanic, wearing greasy overalls. His hands and nails were dark with embedded black oils. The small exam room was filled with strong odors of gasoline and oil. He was hiccupping frequently, about every ten seconds, and could barely get out a few words between hiccups. Between each effort to speak, he gasped for air and groaned. He had been hiccupping continuously for four days and had not slept in the past twenty-four hours. He had lost six pounds and looked near exhaustion. He held onto his rib cage with both arms in an attempt to splint the chest wall pain. The man was in agony, asking for relief.

"Just put me out of this," he kept saying. "Knock me out."

He had tried every folk remedy, to no avail. He had swallowed handfuls of sugar. He had held his breath as long as he could. He had pulled on his tongue and described trying to drink out of a glass from the opposite side of the glass. He had even breathed gasoline fumes, thinking this would knock him out. He wanted me to give him enough drugs to produce unconsciousness so he could sleep.

After taking his medical history and doing a brief physical exam, I could hardly wait to examine the man's ears. The title of the article I had just finished reading was "Hiccups Associated with Hair in the External Auditory Canal—Successful Treatment by Manipulation."

With some anticipation, I looked into the man's left ear, and there it was—a long black hair embedded against the eardrum. I could not believe what I was seeing. I had just read two case reports of chronic hiccups accompanied by a hair on the eardrum. In both cases, hiccups were relieved by removing the hair. Here I was an hour later encountering what I had just read. I took a cotton swab and pulled the hair away from the eardrum. The hiccups stopped abruptly and did not recur. It seemed miraculous. The man sank back on the exam table, exhausted. He repeated over and over, "Thank you. Thank you. Thank you."

He must have thought I was some kind of magical wizard. I felt like one.

The hair on my neck stood up and my heartbeat quickened. I had goose bumps on both arms. I leaned back in my chair in complete awe of what had just happened. For a brief moment I thought of divine intervention. Later I rejected that notion. I could not imagine an all-powerful God orchestrating the delivery of a medical journal to a second-year medical resident just in time for him to be ready to see a man within the next hour with hiccups from a hair on the eardrum. Somehow I don't think it works quite that way.

What exactly is a hiccup? Hiccups consist of an intermittent, spasmodic contraction of the diaphragm and other muscles used for breathing. Since they are often associated with eating, they may serve as a mechanism to dislodge food from the esophagus.

So how does a hair against the eardrum produce hiccups? The nerve paths are complicated. Apparently irritation of the eardrum can produce hiccups, as in this and the other three reported cases, by sending signals to the diaphragm. The occurrence of coughing that occurs occasionally when cleaning the ear canal with cotton-tipped swabs is probably produced by the same neurological connections.

The timing of my reading the journal and then seeing the man with hiccups within such a short time proved to be all the more uncanny, because in the forty-six years since, I have not seen another patient with hiccups due to a hair pressing on the eardrum. In 1982, there was a report in the literature of another case in a twenty-seven-year-old man. I can find only these three cases in the medical literature. The man I saw in 1961 would make four cases.

I often hear physician colleagues tell me they read something new about a disease in a medical journal and within a few days, they see an example of it in their practice. I have no explanation for such occurrences. All I know is such things do happen. Sometimes evidence is just handed to medical detectives.

Chapter Six

A Paralysis of Pregnancy

There was some urgency when I got the call from Mobile, Alabama. Dr. Ford Gitland was referring a patient to me in Birmingham, where I was on the medical faculty of the University of Alabama in Birmingham (UAB).

"You will never believe this. Got a patient here who gets paralyzed every time she gets pregnant. We need you to take her."

Ford Gitland was a former resident who had been in practice for six or seven years. He went on to tell me that the patient was now seven months into her third pregnancy. In her two previous pregnancies, she had developed extreme weakness and a fast heartbeat (ventricular tachycardia was the rhythm). Both babies died in utero at the seventh and eighth months. Her blood potassium level was extremely low at 1.1. (The normal range is 4.0 to 6.0.)

I had never seen a patient with a blood potassium that low. My mind began to whirl around possible causes in a pregnant woman.

Gitland said, "She is completely paralyzed and on a ventilator. Can you take her?" I told him to send her on with IV potassium running.

Around four o'clock that afternoon, they called me from the ER. Tonya Childs had just arrived by ambulance. Tonya was a twenty-three-year-old unmarried African American. She lived out in the country on a cotton farm. Her family were sharecroppers and were very poor.

When I saw her, she could not lift either arm but was beginning to be able to move her feet. She could not talk because of the tube in her trachea. She appeared mentally alert and could follow simple commands. Her pulse rate was fast at 130, with a ventricular tachycardia rhythm by EKG. Fetal heart sounds were present, but there were no fetal movements. Charles Quill, my obstetrician colleague, met me in the ER and agreed to take Tonya on the obstetrical service as his patient, with me as a medical consultant.

Within a few hours we found that Tonya's urine potassium was also quite low. Over the next three days, after infusion of large amounts of IV potassium, Tonya regained the use of her arms and legs. Her heartbeat returned to normal. With the ventilator removed, she gave a completely normal medical history except for the paralysis and weakness that occurred with each of her three pregnancies.

The cause for the combination of low blood potassium and low urine potassium was a mystery. This usually meant the patient was either vomiting and losing potassium through the stomach, or it meant she had previously had diarrhea and was losing potassium in her stools. Tonya strongly denied either vomiting or diarrhea. Laxative abuse is a common cause of low blood potassium, but she denied any laxative use. She also had not taken any diuretics that would have produced prior loss of potassium in her urine. All we knew was that she had lost a lot of potassium somehow. We needed more detective work.

I was in the medical clinic when they called me from the hospital to tell me Tonya's "auntie" wanted to see me. Lula Childs was a large black woman who appeared to be in her seventies. She had come on the bus from Mobile. When I got to Tonya's room, she called me to come into the hall with her, out of Tonya's hearing. She handed me a one-quart milk carton filled with light gray dirt.

"I think you need to know that Tonya eats a lot of this clay," Lula Childs said. "Tonya don't want me telling you this. But I got to thinking. I thought to myself, maybe this clay got something to do with her weakness."

Lula Childs told me that eating clay was a common practice for pregnant women in her area of Alabama. Most ate just small amounts, but Tonya ate almost a full quart every day or two.

"There is something about being pregnant makes you want to eat clay. Got that sweet taste to it." Auntie Lula went on and on about clay-eating habits.

I raced down to the chemistry lab. We cut the clay into serial dilutions with water and found no potassium in the clay. We did not expect to find any. What I wanted to know was how much potassium the clay would bind up, or "chelate." Chelation is a well-known chemical reaction for many substances. We added increasing amounts of potassium to the clay dilutions and found that the clay could tightly bind huge quantities of potassium, thus blocking its absorption from the intestines. This was the first time I had encountered a clay eater. The mystery was solved by Auntie Lula. Tonya ate enough clay to bind and remove huge quantities of potassium from her body and excrete it in her stools.

Clay eating is well known in the South, particularly among African Americans. Some women, when pregnant, enjoy the slightly sweet taste of the clay. Some get a craving for it when pregnant. The clay is composed of diatomaceous earth deposited over eons of sedimentation in the prehistoric seas. These tiny organisms, diatoms, take up carbon dioxide from the air and settle out as clay after they die. As clay, if ingested, they become powerful chelating agents for potassium and other inorganic salts.

During slavery days, death often occurred in clay eaters. It was reported as *cachexia Africanus* in the medical journals of the early 1800s. The victims wasted away to death, often paralyzed.

Potassium deficiency had not yet been discovered.

As with some of the other medical detective stories, a member of the family, Auntie Lula, provided the essential clue—a milk carton of clay.

Chapter Seven

A Sudden and Unexplained Epidemic in a School

Judy Carson rose early on that Thursday morning, November 12. After getting her master's degree in English, she had come back to teach tenth-grade English in her hometown's high school. The class's lesson for the day was to be Elizabeth Barrett Browning's love sonnets.

Fred Harris peddled his bicycle toward the high school after finishing his paper route. His thoughts were focused on the homecoming football game the following day. Fred stopped at the local doughnut and coffee shop on his way.

Betsy Bird was also up early again, reading the sonnets of the coming day's English lesson with Miss Carson. Betsy was an all-A student and one of Miss Carson's favorites.

Judy Carson stopped by the principal's office on the way toward her classroom for the first period of the day. By the time she got to the classroom, all the students were in their seats, jabbering and talking loudly to each other. Miss Carson signaled for silence and walked to her desk.

As she approached her desk, she noted a "foul, gasolinelike odor." The internal events in Judy Carson's mind and body suddenly became real and acute and serious. Her first thought was that the gas was poisonous. Before she could have another thought or give any consideration to an alternative explanation for the odor, the physiology of her body responded in the way it would and should in the face of a life-threatening poisonous fume. What happened to Miss Carson was real. The fumes burned into her nose and sinuses. Judy Carson thought she was dying. Her unconscious mind took control of all functions as Miss Carson stumbled toward the doorway of the classroom. She yelled out, "Get out! Poison gas!" It was her last memory until she woke in the local hospital emergency room, along with ninety-eight other students and staff of the school. Miss Carson, as she fell to the floor, noted an excruciating headache, nausea, a pain in the pit of her stomach, and a sudden shortness of breath. She lost consciousness and was unaware of the stampede of her students as they emptied the classroom, jumping over her body.

Betsy Bird was sitting in the front row, just in front of Miss Carson's desk. She watched Judy Carson approach the desk and then gasp for air, rush toward the door, and fall to the floor. Betsy quickly rose from her seat to approach Miss Carson when she noted an unusual sweet smell. It was strong and burned her nostrils. She too developed shortness of breath and fell to the floor, unconscious.

Fred Harris was now standing in his desk seat at the back of the room. He saw Miss Carson fall, then he saw Betsy Bird fall, followed by five more girls in the front of the room. And then the room emptied. Fred did not smell any odor. He was completely puzzled by what he had witnessed.

Miss Carson's students spread out down the halls, calling into the other classrooms as they ran. "Get out! Poisonous gas! Get out!"

Within a few moments, Mr. Howard Noet, the principal, came over the public address. "Everyone out of the building. This is a fire drill. Everyone out of the building."

Then he kept saying over and over, "Walk slowly, do not run, walk slowly, do not run."

His words were futile. All thirty-six classrooms emptied into the halls in a chaotic mass and out onto the lawn in front of the school. In a few minutes two ambulances arrived and carried off the unconscious bodies of Miss Carson and four students to the emergency room. The ambulances would make eight more trips that morning.

A total of one hundred people would be seen and examined in the local emergency room that day. Eighty of these were students and nineteen were faculty. There was also one parent who happened to be in the school building. Thirty-five people were admitted to the hospital for overnight stays.

All of the physical examinations and lab work of the one hundred affected were normal. All recovered, but several continued to have headaches and residual symptoms.

Mr. Noet closed the school immediately and canceled the football game for Friday night. The police, fire department, several state health department professionals, and state officials of the Occupational Safety and Health Administration (OSHA) made inspections of the buildings and grounds. None could detect any environmental problem, so the school was reopened on Monday, November 16.

On Tuesday, November 17, several students reported severe symptoms requiring ambulance transportation to the emergency room. That day seventy-one persons went to the emergency room with symptoms they thought were associated with exposure to the school. Again, the school was closed, and Mr. Noet launched a full investigation, calling in federal, state, and other authorities to conduct extensive environmental and epidemiologic investigations.

Over the next month, the affected group was interviewed and blood and urine samples were collected. The samples were analyzed for a large number of toxic gases and chemicals. Air samples from the school, along with extensive sampling of the pipes, air conditioning, and other systems, were examined for a long list of toxic materials and gases. None were found. The search for toxic compounds was extended into the surrounding grounds and even into several local caves. Again no toxic materials were found.

Officials from the Centers for Disease Control and Prevention (CDC), the state department of health, and the Preventive Medicine Department of Vanderbilt University joined forces to conduct extensive studies of the epidemic.

The epidemiological studies revealed that girls and women were affected more than males. Those affected most often saw someone who had already been affected, or they had talked to someone who was affected. Nearly all of the affected individuals reported smelling a peculiar odor. The most telling finding was the extreme variation in the descriptions of the odor. There was no uniformity in the descriptions. Some thirty different words were used to describe the odors.

After all of the investigations, the professional investigators agreed that the epidemic was one most accurately labeled as "mass psychogenic illness."

Mass psychogenic illnesses have been known and reported for over six hundred years. There is an extensive literature on the subject. The term, while accurate, is not kindly accepted by those affected. The term "psychogenic" has the connotation that the illness is "all in the mind" or that it is not real, even made up. The mind-body dichotomy, so embedded in our culture, is at the root of the difficulty in understanding this malady. This dichotomy says a disease is either in the body or it is in the mind. The dichotomy rejects the notion that humans are one integrated organism, with no actual separation of mind from body.

Once a belief has been adopted by a person, the whole organism accepts this belief, whether it is based in consensus reality or not. No matter how strange or irrational, we are controlled by our beliefs, whatever they may be. If one truly believes that he or she is breathing a poisonous gas, the body will react as if it were breathing the gas. The chain of physiological reactions will follow. These are not imagined. Not made up. Not "all in the mind." These reactions are measurable and real. If the belief calls for flight, there will be flight in the physiology of the body. If the belief calls for fight, there will be fight.

Miss Carson really had all the symptoms she reported, and she really did fall out and faint. So did all the other students and faculty who followed her in the cascade of the epidemic. Once the mind fires off the malevolent thought or belief, the body's reaction is immediate and, in a curious manner, appropriate for the belief.

The mass psychogenic epidemics serve to illustrate the extreme power of human thoughts and beliefs. The phenomenon is well known in the military, where one fainting by a soldier on parade in hot weather will be followed by an epidemic of faintings, sometimes in the dozens. Almost always, there is line-of-sight transmission. One soldier faints, the next one sees the faint and faints, another sees that faint, and on and on. Line-of-sight transmission is one of the characteristics of a psychogenic epidemic.

Also in the military, there may be one heat stroke followed by witnesses who are feeling the heat, then fall over in unconsciousness, believing they are having a heat stroke. One actual heat stroke can generate many other losses of consciousness to follow.

It is unfortunate that the term "psychogenic" has taken on the negative, even pejorative meanings that it has. In those individuals with lingering symptoms following such epidemics, there can be a tendency to insist that the illness and symptoms are "real." Then the futile process of trying to prove they are really ill with some disease can begin. As Nortin Hadler has pointed out, "If you have to prove you are ill, you can't get well."

There is no easy or ready answer for dealing with these epidemics when they occur. A search for an environmental toxin, especially in these days of terrorism, is certainly justified. However, the negative outcomes will reinforce some to believe there is a cover up or that some toxin has been missed.

One expert in the field states, "The challenge is to convey the scientific reality without being seen as blaming or demeaning the victims."

Even though the nature of the illnesses may be solved, we do not have enough information about the correct way to manage mass psychogenic epidemics at the present time. Even after careful detective work, they remain as mysteries of the mind.

There is one medical illness that is not taught in medical schools or in residencies. It is not listed in the index of any of the major medical textbooks, yet it is quite common. Between 1973 and 1993, there were forty-five epidemics of mass psychogenic illnesses reported from across the globe.

The recent epidemic of Tourette-like syndrome (involuntary jerking of the body) in teenage girls in upper New York State is an example of the illness.

Chapter Eight

Two Cases of Pneumonia: Two Different Causes

Case 1

Susan Swenson and her husband, Fred, ran a feed-and-seed store across the street from their home. Collierville was a small town, like many where the edge of town blends into the surrounding countryside. The Swensons' home and store were part town and part farm.

Fred ran the business end of the store. Susan kept the books. About five o'clock in the afternoon, Susan developed high fever and a shaking chill. Fred immediately put Susan in the truck and headed into the nearby city hospital emergency room. She was put on nasal oxygen. Chest x-rays showed pneumonia in both lower lobes of her lungs. Antibiotics were started and Susan was admitted to the hospital. This would be her third bout of pneumonia in a year.

Dr. Anthony Richards, Susan's doctor, was completely puzzled by the recurring pneumonia. As soon as Susan was able, he ordered a complete workup of her pulmonary function. Dr. Richards suspected some chronic lung condition, such as chronic bronchitis or chronic obstructive pulmonary disease (COPD). Susan had never smoked, adding to the puzzle. All of her lung function tests were normal, ruling out any underlying chronic condition that might make her prone to recurrent infections.

33

Richards then ordered a full workup of Susan's immune system, including a test for HIV/AIDS. Susan at first refused the HIV test, but Richards insisted on pursuing any possible underlying cause.

Fred said, "Does Dr. Richards think we are some IV-drugged-up, sex-crazed hippies?" After Fred calmed down, both agreed to the AIDS test. They were greatly relieved when the test came back negative. All of the other immune tests were normal.

Richards began to wonder if there was some tumor in the trachea or bronchus that was partially obstructing airflow and thus setting the stage for recurrent pneumonias. The bronchoscopy was normal and ruled out that remote possibility. The clues for the cause of the recurring illness remained hidden.

By the next day, the pneumonia had cleared rapidly, and Susan was getting ready to be discharged. Dr. Richards, still baffled by the recurring nature of the pneumonia, called in Dr. Allen Kaiser, an infectious disease specialist. Dr. Kaiser was well known for his ability to tease out histories and explanations for obscure infectious and other diseases. He had been known to inspect people's homes and find clues to other infections, once uncovering the history of cleaning a sick rabbit as the cause of tularemia (rabbit fever) in an elderly woman. Dr. Kaiser was at his best with finishing unsolved clinical puzzles. He could find and fit together pieces in complex illnesses.

Just as Dr. Kaiser entered the room of Susan Swenson, her husband, Fred, came in with her suitcase. Kaiser began his systematic exploration of the history of Susan's past health: her early childhood, her adolescence, the birth of her two healthy daughters, and the subsequent birth of three grandsons—all healthy. Kaiser seemed to be exploring all areas of Susan's life. Like many medical detectives, he knew the life narrative of the patient often led to an understanding of the medical disease. He knew that medical diseases rarely arise *de novo*, out of nowhere.

Knowing the Swensons lived in a small-town, rural setting, Kaiser began asking about possible inhalants.

"Any exposure to cotton lint? Ever worked in a cotton mill?"

"No," Susan answered. Kaiser ruled out cotton lint.

"Do you have a silo on the farm?"

"No." Kaiser ruled out silo-fillers disease.

"Do you handle any wool?"

"No, why do you ask?"

"Don't want to miss wool-gatherer's disease. That's anthrax," Kaiser answered.

Kaiser continued down a long list of questions about exposures of all sorts. For every possibility, he got a negative answer.

After some more time on previous health and illnesses, he turned to the present. "Take me through a typical day in your life. Start with waking and take me through to bedtime," he instructed Susan.

Susan told the story of her life with Fred and their plans to own and operate the feed-and-seed store. She told how she kept the books and sent out the bills. She kept the books at one desk and did the billing and ordering at the two other desks in the back of the store. Some days she did not go to the store, and other days she might spend most of the day in the store.

As Susan told her story, Fred suddenly became animated and interrupted Susan.

"Wait," Fred said, "Tell him about the overhead insect spray. Like how it's automatic."

Dr. Kaiser came to full alert. "How's that?"

Fred told him how they installed an automatic insecticide system in the store about a year ago. The spray nozzle in the office area was over only one desk. That desk was the one least used by Susan, and then only when she did the inventory. The odor of the insecticide spray was ubiquitous in the store, so neither Fred or Susan had considered it as a source of harm.

Kaiser explained that most insecticides contain pyrethrin, a known irritant to the skin and airway. He was certain Fred had given the answer to Susan's pneumonia—pyrethrin pneumonia. The Swensons agreed to remove the overhead insect spray and to keep Kaiser informed of Susan's health. A Christmas card later that year told Kaiser that his diagnosis was correct. Susan had no recurrence of her pneumonia.

Case 2

Raymond and Florence Miller spent the month of June in South Florida. Each year they packed their car and began the several-hundred-mile trip. They lived in northern Indiana, so the trip always took them through Nashville. As they left home, Florence became more and more apprehensive. For two years in a row, she had developed a high fever and pneumonia, leading to hospitalization in a Nashville hospital.

As they crossed the border of Tennessee, Florence began to cough. High fever followed. Once again, for the third year in a row, she was sick. They debated about turning around but decided not. At the emergency room of the hospital, Florence's temperature was 103 degrees and she had paroxysms of coughing. Chest x-rays showed bilateral lower lobe pneumonia. She was admitted and started on antibiotics. By the next morning, she was already much improved.

Dr. Allen Kaiser was asked to see Mrs. Miller. What was the cause of this strange recurring pneumonia that seemed to be triggered by travel into Tennessee? Kaiser went down the list of possible air exposures, as he did with the Swensons in case one.

Florence denied all the suggested possibilities. She did not work in a cotton processing plant and had no exposure to wool fibers. Her air-conditioning system at home was new and had been replaced after her first bout of pneumonia. Kaiser wanted to know if she took some new pillow for the car trip? Was there anything new or special about the car they traveled in? Every question or suggested possible source of inhalants drew a blank.

Florence recovered rapidly and was ready for discharge from the hospital in four days. She would continue the antibiotic for another six days in Florida.

As Florence and Raymond were packing their bags, Dr. Kaiser came into the room. It was the first time he had met Raymond Miller. Ever the detective looking for clues, Kaiser started to run the same exposure questions by Mr. Miller. There just had to be something in the air somewhere to produce repeated bouts of pneumonia in such a tight pattern of recurrence. It just could not be coincidence—June trip to Florida, passage along the same highways, onset of cough and fever just inside the Tennessee line. All of this occurred within a twelve-hour time frame of leaving northern Indiana—three years in a row. Kaiser could not in his wildest imagination believe that Tennessee air was toxic to Florence.

Mr. Miller listened carefully to Dr. Kaiser's questions. His face lit up as he interrupted the questions. "You know, I think I've got it," he said.

Miller went into some detail as he told his story. He was manager of a small electronic parts company. In the manufacture of the electronic parts, avoidance of any moisture was essential. The small factory had a special air-conditioning system with high air turnover and air drying. The final step before packing the parts was to include several dozen plastic packets of a powdered drying agent around each of the electronic devices.

Miller said he got the idea to use the powdered packets at home to fight mildew in their summer clothing. Instead of putting the sealed packets in the dresser drawer with the summer clothing, he cut open the packets and spread the desiccating powder into all layers of the clothing. When Florence Miller packed for the trip, she shook out each piece of clothing, inadvertently inhaling some of the powder. The lack of immediate irritation from the dust had removed it as a possible source of the problem from her memory. Something in the powder had set up a delayed irritation and inflammatory response in Mrs. Miller's lungs that led to the delayed infection and pneumonia.

The mystery of the recurring pneumonia was solved. The powder was removed from the drawer and the summer clothing. The next summer, the Millers finally got past Nashville free of pneumonia and enjoyed their vacation in Orlando, Florida.

These two cases were solved by a master medical detective—Dr. Allen Kaiser of Vanderbilt School of Medicine. Both cases were solved by listening, careful questioning, and involving a family member in the search for clues.

Chapter Nine

Under the Bridges of the Cumberland River

There is one story that still haunts me. It happened over fifty years ago when I was a senior in medical school.

I was rotating in the emergency room of Vanderbilt Hospital. In those days, before the American public began stampeding toward high-tech medicine, the emergency room was relatively quiet much of the time. For the most part, the ER was there only for truly life-threatening accidents and trauma. It was during one of the lulls that the young couple appeared.

Miss Quill was the head nurse. It was clear to all who worked there that she was in charge. Her size alone demanded attention—tall, large, and loud. She never spoke softly.

Miss Quill called me to the front desk and handed me the chart of a child. She pointed to a young couple sitting in the waiting area. The woman held a child in her lap. The child was whimpering quietly.

Both the man and the woman appeared to be in their twenties. Both were dressed in ragged clothing. The man wore a wool cap pulled down low on his forehead. The woman had a scarf tied around her head and neck. Both adults emanated dejection and sadness. They hung their heads low and looked down at the floor. They looked totally defeated.

When I introduced myself, they said nothing. I motioned toward the examining room area and suggested they follow me. The body odors in the small exam room were stifling. I wondered when they had last bathed. I had to keep the exam room door opened to get some fresh air.

I could get no answers to my questions. I asked them to undress the child. The woman, whom I assumed to be the mother, began taking off the baby's clothes. The mother started crying. In a moment, she held out the left arm of the child. There it was. On the upper arm circling the midbiceps area was a raw wound oozing pus. The wound was about half an inch wide and it circled the entire arm. It looked like someone had taken a knife and cut a path all the way around the arm. The cut was obviously infected.

"How did this happen?" I asked, thinking the worst possible causes of such abuse.

Both adults looked at me with blank eyes, said nothing, and shook their heads, as if to say, "We have no idea." I got nowhere with my barrage of questions.

"Did you do this? Did someone else do this? Did you see anyone else handle the baby? How long have you noticed this wound?" All I got back were head shakes or single-syllable answers of no.

I began to wonder if this was some sort of strange worm. I had seen pictures of burrowing worms in some of the tropical medicine books.

"Have you been out of the country?"

"No." I knew it was an absurd question, the moment I asked it.

"Have you noticed worms in your house?"

Again, "No."

What on earth could make a completely circular wound on a year-old baby's arm? I went for Miss Quill. I knew she must have seen it all.

Miss Quill came into the room. She was breathing hard from the exertion of the short walk from her desk back to the exam room.

When she looked at the wound, she said immediately, "Oh, I've seen this before." She pulled a tool off the equipment tray, a kind of small hook like dentists use to pry into cavities in the teeth. She inserted the hook deep into the wound in the child's arm and probed around a bit. The child screamed in pain.

Miss Quill pulled what appeared to be a string out of the wound. Then it was obvious. It was a rubber band. Over a long, unknown time, the rubber band had sunk deep into the arm of the baby. It must have slowly cut its way deeper and deeper into the flesh, finally burying itself from sight. For a rubber band to sink that deep into normal flesh must have taken several weeks. Miss Quill cut the rubber band and pulled it out from around the arm. The baby continued screaming and then gradually quieted with jerky breaths for air between her cries.

Miss Quill turned with a vengeance on the two adults. "What kind of parents are you? When is the last time you bathed this child? When is the last time you even saw her body? How could you let this happen? Did you do this on purpose to your own child?" Miss Quill was furious.

Slowly she got a few answers. The couple was homeless. They lived in a cardboard box under one of the bridges across the Cumberland River. They ate garbage. They had no money and both were out of work. They had walked several miles from town out to the hospital. Neither had seen the wound before. The reason they came to the ER was to find out why the baby cried all the time. No one knew how the rubber band got on the arm of the baby.

After the wound was cleaned and dressed, Miss Quill called social services to meet with the couple.

The immediate mystery of a circumferential infected wound in a baby was solved. Like many medical mysteries, that part was easy. The deeper and more tragic mystery, the one that buried itself in my memory for over fifty years, remains. I have not encountered a starker example of how futile medical care really can be. We patch up people and then send them right back into the situation that caused the problem in the first place. Medicine is too often a tragic profession— a first-aid station in a never-ending war zone of human depravity, poverty, and hardship. No medical detective work can solve the crimes of inhumanity.

That couple and that baby were really no better off in the long run after we removed the rubber band. We sent them back to their cardboard box under the bridge across the Cumberland River.

Chapter Ten

Some Things Just Get Under Your Skin

Sam Waffard lived in the country about thirty miles from the city. He had developed a strange illness that prompted repeated admissions to Vanderbilt Hospital.

The only history he gave was that he would notice a strange feeling over his chest and shoulders. Within a few hours he had shaking chills and high fever. Each time he came to the ER, he was admitted. Sam appeared to be a muscular, healthy young man in his early twenties. The only abnormality on physical examination, other than fever, was the finding of air under his skin over the front and back of his chest. The air extended to his shoulders and lower neck. The doctors told him it was called "subcutaneous emphysema."

On each admission, cultures were taken from his blood and from samples of the gas under his skin. No bacterial organism was ever cultured. After the first few admissions, Sam had become famous to the medical residents and the faculty at the medical school. Each resident was determined to become the detective who would find the cause for the curious findings of air under the skin and high fever. Each time Sam was admitted, he began a course of antibiotics. The fever quickly went away and Sam recovered, only to be readmitted several weeks later.

No one had ever seen a case of high fever and spontaneous sub-cutaneous emphysema. Air under skin of the chest is well known to occur in some patients with rib fractures or penetrating wounds to the chest wall. Sam had neither. Air under the skin can also occur around surgical tracheostomy sites in the neck, where the air from the airway dissects out under the skin of the neck. Sam had never had a tracheostomy or any operation on his neck.

Cases as unusual as Sam's nearly always get presented at the weekly grand rounds at the medical school. The case is presented by the resident, and the findings are discussed by the faculty. Sam's case had been presented several times, but no one had come up with an explanation for the combination of air under the skin, infection, and fever. Various members of the faculty had suggested many different causes for the air to accumulate under the skin. Was there some hidden connection between his trachea and the skin? Or maybe there was a connection between his esophagus and the skin. Could there be a connection between his throat and the skin? All of these were excluded by radiographic studies. One faculty suggested that the infecting agent, which had never been cultured, might be some strange gas-forming bacillus. That possibility had never been tested, since none of the cultures grew bacteria for examination. Maybe this was a new disease.

There was one member of the faculty who was famous for making difficult diagnoses — for solving medical mysteries, which Sam's case had become. Dr. Rudolph Kampmeier was known as a diagnostician without a peer, and he was called to see and examine Sam.

Dr. Kampmeier's most recognized ability was taking the best histories around. If there was a history to be obtained, Kampmeier was the one who could get it. One time an elderly couple was admitted; both had syphilis of the aorta. Both were missionaries, so the house staff were embarrassed to ask about the origins of the syphilis in this pious husband and wife. Aortic syphilis is a late stage of the disease, often taking fifteen or more years to develop after the primary infection. Dr. Kampmeier, alone, approached the elderly male missionary to get the full story.

The old man told Dr. Kampmeier that he and his wife had been missionaries in the jungles of Southeast Asia. One day, while walking through the jungle, he came across a young native girl. Before long they had sexual intercourse, and a week later he developed a sore on his penis, the primary lesion of syphilis. He told Kampmeier that was his only transgression from his wife. If a doctor can get that kind of history from an elderly missionary, he probably can get any kind of history from anybody. Kampmeier had that reputation.

Late one night, when all of the lights were out on the sixteen-bed ward, Dr. Kampmeier quietly approached the bed of Sam. The head nurse overheard Dr. Kampmeier say, "Now, son, it is time you told someone the whole truth." No one heard any of the rest of the conversation.

Here is the story Sam told Dr. Kampmeier that night:

Sam lived on a farm in a remote section of the next county. His father ran a gas station where Sam worked part time. (Sam called it a "filling station.") Sam's girl friend, Elena, lived half a mile down the road. Often they met at night and sneaked into a back room in the gas station, where they enjoyed sex with each other. This, however, was not the usual kind. Elena had persuaded Sam to let her pump air under his skin with a bicycle pump. She bit a small hole in his shoulder and inserted the metal needle of the pump under his skin and pumped in air. The air dissected under the skin until it covered his chest. Sam told Dr. Kampmeier that Elena liked the crunchy feel of the air under the skin so he just went along with her. On some occasions the contamination of the needle with saliva caused infection. Sam learned to come to the hospital and get antibiotics when that happened.

No one knows what instructions Dr. Kampmeier gave him, but Sam was never admitted again. No one ever knew what led Dr. Kampmeier to know Sam needed to make a confession.

I wonder how many medical mysteries would be solved by full confessions.

The Mystery Is Not What, But Why

Twenty-six-year-old Veronica was on the faculty of a nearby junior college nursing school. Veronica looked and dressed like a fashion model. She radiated cheerfulness in our first meeting, smiling even when she described her past serious illnesses. The dean of the nursing school had referred her to see me.

Veronica was covered in bruises. Some looked superficial, but others looked deep and purple—the kind I have always associated with serious clotting disorders or with blood diseases like leukemia. It did not take great detective work to find the clues for Veronica's problems.

The superficial bruises were all paired in a butterfly pattern, the tell-tale sign of self-infliction. Pinching the skin to the point of bruising always leaves a pair of bruises resembling a butterfly. The other giveaway in self-inflicted bruises is their complete absence between the shoulder blades, an area that cannot be reached by the person's fingers. Veronica had been causing her own paired bruises. But what about the deep purple bruises?

Veronica had grown up the only child of missionaries in Africa and told harrowing stories of one injury after another. As I was examining her eyes, she casually mentioned that her left eye had been sliced when a knife slipped in her hand. She said the vitreous liquid from her eye ran down her cheek and she had to hold the eyeball in place with her hand until they got to the nearest village. She said the missionary doctor sewed the eye back in place. When I questioned the absence of a scar she told me what a wonderful surgeon the doctor had been. She waved off my question, responding in a bored tone of voice, as if to say, why did you even ask that stupid question?

She told some dramatic story with nearly every organ I palpated or discussed. Her heart had been inflamed when she was a child, and she had nearly died in the jungle clinic. She had had some rare pulmonary fungus that had finally healed. She had vomited blood and had blood in her stools, as well as in her urine. She had been in shock from blood loss from a jeep accident in the jungles of the Congo. Both legs had been broken when she fell out of a tall tree. All of these stories were told in a calm, nearly bored tone of voice.

I stopped passing comments and just listened to one story after another. I think I said something like, "It's a wonder you are still alive."

Concerned with the deep purple bruises, I admitted her to the hospital to work up her blood clotting and coagulation status. In those days, 1977, admissions to hospitals were readily available. Hospitals provided wonderful opportunities to observe and to get to know patients. Her clotting time was greatly prolonged, as were the other clotting factors, all tests pointing toward a circulating anticoagulant. She had taken or injected some chemical to inhibit clotting. Both defects were corrected in the test tube with protamine sulfate, the agent known to reverse heparin effect. (Heparin is the anticoagulant used to treat clotting problems such as deep vein thromboses.) Veronica had done two things; she was injecting herself with heparin, and she was also pinching herself to produce smaller paired superficial bruises.

I called in my psychiatric associate, Harry Abram, to help. He and I had often discussed patients who inflict diseases on themselves—so-called factitious or factitial diseases. In Veronica's case, we would label her as someone with the Munchausen syndrome, named after a Baron von Munchausen, an eighteenth-century aristocrat in Germany. The baron was not ill, but he had a reputation of telling tall tales. During the nineteenth century, stories about his fantastical adventures were circulated in Germany. Thus, his name was assigned to describe those patients who go from hospital to hospital telling tall tales of their self-inflicted illnesses. Veronica's "illness" was an example of the Munchausen syndrome.

Abram and I had been waiting for the next such case to come along. He wanted to see if he could make any psychiatric sense out of the patient. At that time, and it still may be true, there were no factitial patients in the literature who had been carefully observed or treated in psychiatry over a long period. Harry was interested in uncovering the psychodynamics of such patients. This was going to be a first for both of us.

After we corrected the heparin effect in Veronica and all of her clotting factors were back to normal, I discharged her from the hospital. We had a clear understanding with her that she was to see both me and Harry Abram in follow-up (or so we thought). I had been very direct in telling her that I knew of the heparin injections and the danger associated if she continued doing that. Even after discharge, she continued to deny that she had dosed herself. I felt uncomfortable continuing to see her, but I had made a pact with Abram to follow one such patient with him—no matter what.

The next time I saw Veronica was about a month later. She had a huge abscess on her upper outer left arm, near the shoulder. She said she had been letting her student nurses practice injections on her, and obviously one of the students must have broken sterile technique and infected her arm. I called the dean of the nursing school and inquired about the student nurses using instructor's arms for practice sites. She called back to tell me that had not happened. Again Veronica denied any self-infliction. I called Abram and suggested we terminate our pact. He insisted that he was beginning to make headway, despite the abscess occurrence. Once more I reluctantly agreed to continue to follow Veronica medically.

Within a few weeks after the abscess had been drained, Veronica came into the emergency room. The physician on call admitted her with a temperature of 104 degrees. The next morning when I saw her, her temperature was 102 degrees with a normal pulse rate of 76. The low pulse did not fit with the fever. It should have been higher.

I called the nurse and we checked the temperature under observation and it was 98.8 degrees. Obviously, Veronica had heated the thermometer. Again she denied it, saying she had no explanation for the sudden drop in fever. Again I called Abram, and he urged me to continue, saying something like, "Well, you didn't expect we would make quick progress on such a tough clinical problem, did you?"

Over the next two months Abram saw Veronica weekly and reported to me that he was establishing strong rapport but still had no insights into the psychodynamics or the origins of Veronica's need to inflict disease on herself. He had no explanation as to the psychological origins of her problem.

The next time I saw Veronica, she was complaining of extreme weakness. She was as pale as the sheets she lay on. She was anemic, with low hemoglobin levels. I admitted her to the hospital. With her rapid pulse, she showed signs of obvious acute blood loss. Her blood smears also showed evidence of iron deficiency, an indication of chronic blood loss. I began to transfuse her. She told me her menses had been extremely heavy, and that was why she showed blood loss anemia.

That afternoon as I entered Veronica's room, I found her running blood from the IV tubing from her arm back into the trash can by her bedside. In the face of severe anemia, she was continuing to bleed herself via the tubing. That was it. I called Abram, and we transferred Veronica to the psychiatric unit. When she was finally discharged, I gave her written notice that she must find another medical doctor, and I resigned from her care. Abram said he would continue to see her for psychiatric care.

Several months went by. Abram told me she had stopped coming to see him. Several more months went by, when I got a call from a hospital in Atlanta. They told me Veronica has been admitted with severe anemia. She told the doctor there that I had been treating her for acute leukemia. She also told tall tales of her many illnesses and injuries. I shared my failed experiences with Veronica and wished him more luck than I'd had in treating her.

At that time in my practice, I was deeply captivated by two of the most gripping fantasies young physicians can have. The first of these is an unrealistic sense of omnipotence. Veronica's self-inflicted damage stood in the face of my false sense of omnipotence. Her repeated self-destructive acts stemmed from her inner problems, not from any impotence on my part. However, I failed to understand that at first. The second intense fantasy of many young physicians is the belief that they can rescue every single patient in distress, no matter what the circumstances really are. This rescue fantasy is also unrealistic and impossible in many situations. I also failed to understand the need in myself to rescue others.

Of all of the patients with medical mysteries, I found those with factitial or self-inflicted diseases to be the most difficult. Finding the self-infliction was easy. Helping to correct the behavior was difficult.

Even as I made adjustments to my fantasies of omnipotence and rescue, I still found them difficult for me to accept. I did not see that the only language such patients have is one of self-infliction. I never learned to make the translations of their language into one that I could understand and accept.

There are doctors who have had success in helping people with self-inflicted diseases. Dr. Marc Feldman records such experiences in his book, *Playing Sick* (New York: Routledge, 2004).

The medical mystery with self-inflicted disease is not *what* these people do to harm themselves, but *why*. That mystery has not yet been solved.

Chapter Twelve

Some Diseases Are Like Serial Killers

Sometimes diseases are like serial killers. They strike in isolation.

Victim One
Anderson Donavan
Admitted to City Hospital
12:30 P.M. September 29, 1963
Died October 5, 1963

At 12:30 P.M. on Sunday, September 29, 1963, Anderson Donavan, a forty-seven-year-old white man, appeared in the emergency room of the city hospital. On awakening that morning, he had noted dizziness and difficulty focusing on near objects. He said that when looked at single objects, he saw three. The dizziness increased until he felt the room was spinning around. Nausea and severe vomiting soon followed, along with an intense sore throat.

The medical resident who saw Donavan said the man did not look sick, but a blood pressure of 70/50 induced him to admit the patient to the city hospital. The physical examination showed widely dilated pupils that responded poorly to light. Eight hours after admission, he suffered a cardiac arrest. With closed chest compression, his heartbeat was reestablished. However, he remained on a ventilator for a week, completely unresponsive to all stimuli. Donavan was pronounced dead on October 5. No autopsy was performed. The admitting diagnosis was "thrombosis of the basilar artery of the brain stem." This incorrect diagnosis would not be corrected until a week after his death.

Victim Two
Fenders Stevens
Admitted to the local Veterans Administration hospital (across town from the city hospital)
September 29, 1963
Died September 30, 1963

Two hours after Donavan (victim one) was admitted to the city hospital on September 29, Fenders Stevens (victim two) was admitted to the Veterans Administration hospital. Donavan and Stevens did not know each other. Stevens, a thirty-seven-year-old white man, was known to be a heavy drinker. Twenty-four hours before admission, he consumed five to six beers. Shortly after the beers, he developed dizziness, difficulty walking, progressive weakness, nausea, and vomiting. He also noted difficulty swallowing and a peculiar sound to his speech. He noted progressive swelling of his abdomen, difficulty urinating, and a dry mouth.

Stevens said, "I ain't never had a drunk like this before. Hell, I think somebody poisoned me."

On examination, his vital signs were all normal. He was alert and well oriented. His pupils were widely dilated and fixed. His speech was nasal. His eyelids drooped, and he had difficulty protruding his tongue. He had severe muscle weakness and could not stand without support. Because of the suspicion of food poisoning, he and his family were questioned about unusual foods or spoiled home-canned products over the past several days. None were recalled.

After admission, Stevens was put on a ventilator because of increasing difficulty breathing. Eighteen hours after admission, Stevens was dead. A postmortem examination failed to reveal any cause for the death. Tissues and blood were frozen for later examination.

54

Victim Three
Annie Mc Andrews
Admitted to Local Hospital One
October 6, 1963
Died October 6, 1963

One day after victim one, Anderson Donavan, died in the city hospital, Annie McAndrews, a fifty-year-old white woman, was admitted to Local Hospital One with severe nausea and vomiting. None of the three victims knew or had any social contact with the other victims. None of the physicians or nurses knew of the deaths of the first two victims.

Annie McAndrews developed severe muscle weakness and respiratory failure. She was dead a few hours after admission to the hospital. There was no diagnosis at the time of her death.

Victim Four
Gregory Frees
Admitted to Local Hospital Two
October 6, 1963

At Local Hospital Two, Gregory Frees, a fifty-four-year-old white man, was admitted with nausea, vomiting, and severe abdominal swelling. X-rays of his abdomen showed large dilated loops of bowel, suggesting intestinal obstruction. At surgery, no obstruction was found, and the abdomen was closed. Postoperatively, he developed profound muscle weakness and increasing respiratory failure from the muscle weakness. He was transferred to Vanderbilt Hospital for ventilator support on October 9.

These four cases occurred in isolation from each other. All developed severe respiratory failure, leading to death in the first three; Frees, victim four, survived. Not until a phone call on October 7 did anyone begin to connect the common thread of these cases; all had been admitted to separate hospitals. The serial killer was about to be identified.

Victim Five
Lawrence Bates
An important phone call
October 7, 1963

On Monday morning, October 7, Lawrence Bates, a fifty-three-year-old white man, phoned the emergency room of Vanderbilt Hospital. In a halting, thick-tongued voice, he asked the medical resident, "What are the symptoms of botulism?" When questioned, Bates said he had just heard a radio broadcast telling of an outbreak of botulism in Knoxville, Tennessee. The outbreak was attributed to consumption of smoked whitefish sold in vacuum-packed plastic bags through a large supermarket chain. Bates said he had eaten some of the fish the evening before and had noted nausea and vomiting that morning, followed by dry mouth, weakness, and difficulty speaking. He was advised to come immediately to the ER.

Bates had a BP of 100/60 and a dilated left pupil (the right eye was sightless due to detached retina). His speech was slurred and nasal. The mouth and tongue appeared dry. There was no muscle weakness. He was admitted with a tentative diagnosis of suspected cerebrovascular accident rather than botulism. The lack of muscle weakness at that time diverted attention away from botulism.

A few hours after Bates was admitted, the family of victim two (Fenders Stevens) called the VA hospital and told the physician that Stevens had eaten the same brand of whitefish implicated in the Knoxville cases of botulism. The word was out, and the association of botulism with smoked whitefish spread across town, the hospitals, the medical community, and the state.

With this new information and despite the lack of muscle weakness, Stevens was given Types A, B, and E botulism antitoxin.

All of the families of victims one, two, three, and four heard of the Knoxville report, and they called to say that the victims had all eaten the smoked whitefish. The diagnosis of botulism was then firmly established from the timing of eating the fish and the symptoms.

Three more patients, within the next two weeks, would be seen with a history of eating the same brand of smoked whitefish and symptoms of botulism. All were given antitoxin to botulism A, B, and

E. All five victims who were given the antitoxin lived and recovered from the illness.

Botulism, the Disease

Botulism is caused by a bacterium that forms spores and secrets a toxin. Types A and B *Clostridium botulinum* usually result from poorly processed home canning. The organism of this outbreak was found to be Type E. Type E comes from poorly processed fish or fish products. Botulism is not caused by an infectious organism that invades the body, even though a bacterium causes the illness. The illness comes from the toxin generated by the bacteria, usually when the bacterium is outside the human body.

In Types A and B botulism, the food often tastes funny or putrid. Such is not the case with Type E, where there is no peculiar taste to the food. In this outbreak, eighteen individuals ate some of the smoked whitefish. Eight of the eighteen developed the disease, for an attack rate of 44 percent. Botulism Type E is sometimes seen in waterfowl around the Great Lakes. The birds eat dead fish that have washed up on the shores. The paralysis starts in the necks of the birds, hence the name "limber neck" for the disease in birds.

Botulism toxin is a neurotoxin, and it blocks the action of the nerves, producing paralysis of all muscles. The muscles of respiration are affected, so the usual mode of death is respiratory failure, just like the first three fatal cases, none of whom received the antitoxin. The toxin is said to be one of the most toxic substances known. Very small amounts have been known to be fatal. The toxin is heat labile, hence cooking temperatures are effective detoxifying procedures.

There is no specific laboratory test for the presence of botulism toxin. The classic symptom complex is the only clue, together with a history of ingesting spoiled processed food or seafood that has spoiled. Serial dilutions of the patient's blood serum can be injected into mice. Death of the mice from small amounts of serum is presumptive evidence for botulism toxin.

There is no specific drug to treat botulism. Type-specific antitoxins are known to be effective treatment in some cases. The antitoxin is prepared by inoculating horses and using the horse's serum for injection into humans. The present available antitoxin combines Type A, B, and E antitoxin.

Like a serial killer who poisons his victims, botulism slipped undetected from one victim to the next, leaving no tell-tale sign. The mystery was solved only from the history of ingesting the poisoned fish.

Chapter Thirteen

Three Years of Diarrhea

Agnes Mayhugh was a twenty-seven-year-old secretary. She told a story of long-standing diarrhea of over three years' duration. Two years earlier she had been admitted to a local hospital for a workup of the problem. The doctors found gallstones, and she'd had her gallbladder removed. The diarrhea continued.

About a year earlier, she had been readmitted to another hospital and had an extensive workup of her gastrointestinal tract with upper and lower endoscopy and several barium studies. A biopsy of her small intestine was done via a swallowed tube. She was told that she might have ulcerative colitis or Crohn's disease in an early phase. The basis for these suggestions of diagnoses was never found in a review of her outside records. The biopsy of her small bowel was normal.

Someone told her she might need to have her colon removed. That is when she was referred to see me. I reviewed all of her outside records, the results of the barium studies of her GI tract, and all of her lab results. Everything was normal.

Agnes had noted no pattern to the occurrences of her diarrhea. I asked that she keep a diary noting the time of each bowel movement, where she was at the time, and a close record of what she had eaten. She kept her diary for three weeks and even tried omitting certain foods and liquids. She noted no effects, but she had noted that the diarrhea was less on the weekends.

In setting up diary keeping with patients, I want them to keep a completely open mind. I don't want to head in either a physical or psychological direction exclusively. I want them to make observations about the substances they are eating and the people they are seeing. Over the next month, she began to notice that her symptoms were worse toward the end of the week.

I had asked her my two favorite questions. Notice how both are open ended:

What are you doing in your life that you should *stop* doing? And,

What are you *not* doing in your life that you should be doing?

I had found that these two highly unspecified questions provoke a deep memory search in patients with symptoms of unknown origin. If you think about the wording of the questions, you will see that they are limitless, and therefore they provoke a search of every aspect of one's life. They call for the patient to look for activities in life that should be stopped or for activities that should be added.

Agnes came back a week early for her next appointment. She blurted out a long story of her boss. He ran an office in a collection company and worked directly for the owner of the company. For over three years, Agnes knew he was embezzling money from the company. He had confronted Agnes on several occasions when he found out that she had discovered the embezzlement. He had involved her sufficiently that she was not entirely free of the crime. For the past year, she had avoided all connections with his theft but remained in conflict over what to do.

Agnes went to night college and needed the income to continue her college work for her degree. If she reported him, he would involve her in the crime, and she would lose her job. If she did not, her sense of guilt and low self-esteem were nearly intolerable.

Even after she told me this story, she said, "But none of that has anything to do with my diarrhea."

I did not see Agnes for several months. When she reappeared in the clinic, she was smiling and laughing with the nurse. I hardly recognized her. She was all dressed up with a new hairstyle. She no longer slumped over but stood erect. She was no longer an unattractive woman. The transformation was remarkable.

She introduced her boyfriend as her fiancé and told me of the upcoming marriage.

She had thought and thought about her situation, and even though she did not think the diarrhea was related to the job and the situation with her boss, she had resigned and reported him to the owner of the company. She said a great weight was lifted from her. In a few weeks, the diarrhea ceased.

She said it took her several weeks to realize how stressed she had been in the job. She said stopping the diarrhea was not the major change she had noted. She said she got her life and spirit back. She thanked me. I wished her and her fiancé the best. I never saw Agnes again after that day.

Over the years I am frequently reminded of how true the old sayings are. "He makes me want to vomit," or "She is a pain in the ass," or "He gives me a headache," or "This job is breaking my back."

Or, as in the case of Agnes, "He makes me have diarrhea."

Some people make us sick if we let them. Bringing the issues into awareness is the first step in the process of healing. I suspect there are many painful medical mysteries that go unsolved because they are buried in toxic relationships. The patients in these situations must become their own detectives.

Chapter Fourteen

The Case of Mrs. Oliver Townwell

Mrs. Townwell was the wife of the owner of a successful insurance agency in a small town in southern Mississippi. Her husband, and even some of her closest acquaintances, called her "Mrs. Townwell." Few people even knew her first name. She always called her husband "Mr. Townwell."

The Townwells had two daughters: Estelle was the older and Juanita, the younger. Both were married, and each had two children, a boy and a girl. Shortly after Juanita's birth, Mrs. Townwell began to develop weakness in her legs. Over the next five years, the weakness progressed until she was confined to a wheelchair.

Mrs. Townwell was seen by many specialists in New Orleans and Memphis, but no one was able to make a diagnosis or suggest treatment. Both daughters bought houses on the same street as Mrs. Townwell so they could be close to their now-paralyzed mother. Every other night the daughters rotated spending the night in their mother's home. Mr. Townwell had moved into a separate bedroom upstairs to provide his bed for the daughters, so they could be in the room with their mother. Mrs. Townwell moved her bed into what had been the family dining room at the front of the house. From that room she had a commanding view of all who passed by on the street.

The only time Mrs. Townwell left her house was to attend the First Baptist Church. Each Sunday at the eleven o'clock service, both daughters, Mr. Townwell, and the other family members accompanied Mrs. Townwell down the aisle to the same seat on the second row of pews. The daughters alternated pushing their mother in the wheelchair. Mr. Townwell always followed in the rear of the small procession of the two daughters, two sons-in-law, and the four grandchildren. The pastor always came down to greet her and say a brief prayer before the service began. Outside the church, there was always a crowd of well wishers, who gathered around Mrs. Townwell's wheelchair. Mrs. Townwell's name had been on the church's prayer list for invalids for over twenty years. After the Sunday service, the family always ate at the Downtown Café. After the meal Mr. Townwell drove Mrs. Townwell home, where she took a long nap each Sunday afternoon. On sunny days, if Mrs. Townwell was strong enough after her nap, they went for a late-afternoon automobile ride into the countryside. Mrs. Townwell always wore her nightgown and bathrobe.

Twenty-three years after Mrs. Townwell was confined to her wheelchair, Mr. Townwell dropped dead in his office. The funeral was held in the First Baptist Church, followed by a graveside service at the Magnolia Cemetery. At the cemetery, when the wheelchair was brought around to the car door for Mrs. Townwell, she waved it away, stood up, and slowly walked to the graveside. There was a humming murmur from the crowd of people. Several moved closer to see her walk to the graveside. Some thought they had witnessed a miracle. The pastor mentioned the miracle in his comments in the following Sunday service.

Mrs. Townwell never used her wheelchair again, and she never discussed or explained her long illness.

Over several years following the death of Mr. Townwell, it became general knowledge in the town that Mr. Townwell had begun a long love affair with his secretary during Mrs. Townwell's second pregnancy, just before the onset of her weakness. The love affair continued until Mr. Townwell's death, over twenty years later.

There are some illnesses so deep and toxic in the soul that they remain mysteries, even after the story is told. Such is the case with Mrs. Oliver Townwell.

Pigs and Pacifiers

Jonathan Roberts sat at his desk in the Tennessee State Department of Health. Roberts had been chief epidemiologist and a master medical detective for twenty-seven years. At first he did not remember seeing anything like the report he had just been handed by Kristen Williams, the young medical student assigned to work with him for the spring. She showed him a list of twelve patients with severe diarrhea and with stool cultures positive for *Yersinia enterocolitica.* The epidemic occurred after Christmas 2001. A dim light went off in his memory.

The bacterium *Yersinia enterocolitica* is an uncommon cause of disease outbreaks in the United States. Of 7,390 food-borne disease outbreaks reported to the Centers for Disease Control and Prevention (CDC) from 1990 through 1999, only five cases were reported to be caused by *Yersinia.* Jonathan Roberts's encyclopedic mind knew those figures just as precisely as he knew the figures for all causes of food-borne illness. Even though it is a rare cause of disease, something from deep inside his brain signaled a recollection about *Yersinia* outbreaks. He was only aware at the time that there was some memory, some experience, some remote activity that was on its way to his consciousness. He knew that he knew; but not what he knew.

Roberts' specialty was food-borne infections. Over the years he had investigated outbreaks of all kinds of diarrhea, nausea, and vomiting from contaminated foods. He spent one summer in a mining camp in California to trace down a remote stream contaminated with *Shigella*. He had located the source of staphylococcal food poisoning in the pastries on board a cruise ship in the Miami harbor. Once, in an outbreak of typhoid fever, he found the food handler who prepared the salads for a banquet of five hundred people. Most of the smaller clusters of infections were from *Salmonella* or *Shigella* organisms, and most were directly traceable to contaminated food handlers. Roberts was passionate about his work and always jumped into investigations with full energy. If the time ever came, he pictured himself as the one who would uncover some alien plot to poison the entire population. He would be the one to uncover a mass terrorist movement to contaminate the entire water supply or infect the milk distribution for a metropolitan area. There was a large dose of the detective in him. And when he saw the *Yersinia* culture results from the stool cultures, he went on full alert. Twelve cases of *Yersinia* would be a record number.

He enjoyed his work in the field, interviewing the victims of the infections, their families, neighbors, and going into their homes and places of work. As soon as he identified the infected cohort, he lined up a matched control group. The selection had to match the infected cohort, but it had to be done randomly. The epidemiological question to be tested necessitated finding the differing behaviors between the infected group and the matched uninfected control group. Over the years he had developed a nearly foolproof system of investigation. He went down a steady list of clues, each one leading him closer to the conclusion and to the identification of the culprit. In outbreaks at schools or in other large groups, he liked to chart the exact seating location of those infected. He demanded to know exactly which tables each server had serviced. He was always looking for patterns or for any clustering that could suggest the source of the infection. He constantly sought the telltale clue that would narrow his search.

Kristen had tallied the information about the recent outbreak of *Yersinia enterocolitica*. The twelve patients were all under the age of one year. None of the families lived close to any of the others, and none knew any of the other families of the infected infants.

None attended the same church. Those with older children did not attend the same school. Human-to-human transmission seemed to be ruled out. The only common denominator was that all twelve infants were black.

The twelve infants had been ill between mid-November and the tenth of February. Six cases became ill within a week of Christmas Day. What was it about the holiday season and being black that caused a *Yersinia* infection?

Jonathan Roberts listened carefully. From deep inside his extensive bank of memories, the faint neurological circuit surfaced to consciousness in his brain. All he said was, "Hog-killing time."

Kristen stopped her reporting and looked puzzled. "What made you say that?"

Roberts answered, "Christmastime, all black patients, and cold weather. All that equals only one thing: hog-killing time."

Questionnaires were circulated to the affected families, and telephone interviews were conducted. A control group of infants was randomly selected from patients matched for age, gender, race, and date seen during the same time period at the same hospital emergency room. Compared to 35 percent of the controls, 100 percent of the infected infants' families had prepared chitterlings within four days of the onset of the diarrhea.

Chitterlings (nearly always pronounced "chitlins") are prepared by cleaning hog intestines, scraping the lining of the intestines, and removing fecal material and fat. Each of the infected families had cleaned between ten and eighty pounds of hog intestines. The cleaning was done in the kitchen sink in the homes. All infected infants had been in the kitchen during the cleaning process. All infants had been contaminated by splatter onto milk bottles or pacifiers or by direct splatter onto the infant.

The intestines, after washing, are then boiled and most likely sterilized. None of the infected infants had eaten chitterlings.

Jonathan Roberts then recalled similar reported epidemics of *Yersinia* infections due to contamination of infants from cleaning hog intestines, but this epidemiological recollection had not triggered his utterance of "hog-killing time." That association came from deeper memories of his youth on a farm in South Georgia, where

Thanksgiving and the arrival of cold weather announced it was hog-killing time—in time for "chitlins" at Christmas. And if the cleaning of the intestines was not done with care and away from contact with infants, it would also be time for *Yersinia* infections.

Chapter Sixteen

The Nurse Solves the Mystery

Mrs. Beatrice Woosley was admitted to 3West of the university hospital with an initial diagnosis of kidney stones.

On her last admission, five weeks earlier, pieces of a stone were recovered from her strained urine and analyzed. The stones were found to contain xanthine. Word quickly circulated among the biochemically oriented faculty of the renal division that a patient with xanthinuria had been found. This extremely rare disorder attracted the attention of the equally biochemically oriented chief of medicine. Beatrice Woosley was then called for readmission to the hospital. The faculty planned a series of special studies and a grand rounds conference to discuss xanthinuria and xanthine kidney stones. Among the faculty there was excitement and anticipation for the upcoming grand rounds. No one had ever seen a patient with a xanthine kidney stone.

Ordinarily xanthine is converted to uric acid and excreted in the urine. People with xanthinuria lack the enzyme that makes this chemical conversion. Xanthine accumulates in the blood and forms deposits, or stones, in the kidney. Like uric acid stones, xanthine stones do not show up on x-rays of the abdomen. This x-ray–invisible state explained the repeated absence of visible stones on x-rays of Beatrice Woosley's kidneys.

This was Beatrice Woosley's fifth admission in three months. She appeared even more frequently in the ER with severe pain from renal colic, each time requiring large amounts of morphine or Demerol for relief.

The purpose of Mrs. Woosley's readmission was to collect more stone fragments for additional chemical analysis and study. On admission, Beatrice Woosley again complained of severe pain on the right side of her back. She said that the pain radiated from the back down into her pubic area—a classic pattern of the pain from passing a kidney stone.

"I got to have something. This pain is killing me," she cried. Each time the nurses gave her morphine, only to have her scream out with more pain after only a few hours.

After admission, she was asked to urinate into a container that had a gauze cover. The gauze strained the urine so that any stone fragment would be caught on the gauze. Sure enough, Beatrice soon produced several small fragments of stones that were rushed to the laboratory for analysis.

On the day after admission, Dr. Joseph Conrad, the medical resident, was called by the nurse to come immediately to Mrs. Woosley's room. The nurse told the young doctor that she had walked into Mrs. Woosley's room to find her sitting on the floor, bent over the urine container. She was picking her gums to produce blood, which she was dripping into the urine container. Patients with kidney stones usually have traces of blood in their urine. Mrs. Woosley was making sure there was some blood in her urine.

The nurse jerked the picking device from Mrs. Woosley's hand and discovered it was a pecan shell. Mrs. Woosley had been faking kidney stone pain in order to maintain her addiction to morphine. She did not have kidney stones but was malingering in order to get her drugs. She had used pecan shells not only to pick her gums, but also to masquerade as kidney stones. She had no idea that pecan shells are high in xanthine, or that xanthine stones are invisible on x-ray, nor did she have any idea of the biochemical interest she had created in the medical faculty. Unwittingly, she had created the almost perfect medical crime—kidney stone malingering with xanthine-loaded pecan shells.

Self-inflicted diseases come in at least two varieties. In chapter 11, Veronica, the nurse instructor, produced all sorts of inflictions and injuries to herself, seemingly for no reason other than to defeat doctors and attract attention for her exploits.

Beatrice Woosley, on the other hand, had a clear purpose for her malingering. Malingerers are seeking some personal gain. Beatrice wanted morphine.

The grand rounds conference on xanthinuria was cancelled and converted to a conference on drug-seeking behavior. There are just no limits to the creativity of malingerers seeking pain-relieving drugs.

Chapter Seventeen

An Outbreak of Bad Eyes

Dr. Dick Grimes was the senior resident in the ER when the first patient was led into the exam area. He had never seen anything like this. It was one thirty in the morning, and he had just finished suturing a laceration.

The patient, Amy Wock, looked to be in her thirties. Arms stuck out in front of her, she was being led like a blind person into the examining room by her husband. She wore a bathrobe over her nightgown. Her head was covered in a towel as she felt her way into the exam room, to avoid hitting the doorway.

"What happened to you?" Dr. Grimes asked.

"We have no idea," Ted Wock, the husband answered. "When she went to bed around eleven o'clock, after we got home from a dinner, everything was fine. She woke just a few minutes ago and screamed out. Then I saw her eyes...awful." Ted grimaced as he spoke.

Dr. Grimes removed the towel. Both eyelids were swollen tightly shut. The tissue around the eyes was red and severely swollen. Tears were running down Amy's reddened cheeks. She quietly moaned in pain. The skin of the entire face was red like sunburn.

"What is it? What is it?" Amy kept asking.

Dr. Grimes attempted to examine Amy's eyes but could not pull the lids apart to see any of the underlying eyeballs.

"Get the ophthalmology resident down here. Stat," he called out to the nurse.

73

"Good idea," the nurse responded. "Another patient with swollen eyes just arrived out front."

When Dr. Jack Mayes, the ophthalmology resident, finished his exam of Amy Wock, he said, "I know what she has but I have no idea how she got it. She has classic photokeratitis. Photokeratitis is caused by exposure to ultraviolet light. Watching someone arc welding will do it, but she denies being around welding."

Dr. Mayes went back over his questioning. No exposure to arc welding, no tanning beds, and certainly no possibility of snow blindness, which also produces photokeratitis. The source of such intense ultraviolet light striking a stranger in the middle of the night was indeed a puzzle.

Just as Dr. Mayes was finishing his examination of Amy Wock, another woman was led into the waiting room by a man. She was staggering along in her bathrobe, hands out in front. Mr. Wock, waiting outside the exam room, saw the couple and rushed to them.

"I can't believe this. My wife may have the same thing. Are her eyes all swollen?" he asked the stranger.

"Yeah, she woke up in severe pain. What is it?" the stranger asked.

"Don't know, waiting on the doctor to tell me."

Over the course of the night, a total of four patients arrived in the ER with severely swollen eyes, complaining of intense pain, sensitivity to light, and blurry vision. All had gone to bed between ten thirty and eleven thirty the night before. Two were women, and two were men. None of them knew each other. All denied any sort of dust exposure or exposure to any kind of spray. By the next morning, seven more people would seek medical attention for swollen and painful eyes.

After extensive study of the epidemic, the only thing in common for the four patients who came to the ER was their attendance at a fund-raising dinner for a not-for-profit charity. Six hundred people had attended the dinner, held in a large auditorium from six to nine o'clock the previous night.

Eighteen people at the dinner had three or more of the following symptoms: redness, burning or itching, sensitivity to light, a foreign body sensation, tearing, blurred vision, swelling, or red skin on the face. The onset of symptoms occurred within twelve hours of the dinner. There were two people who were wearing ultraviolet radiation protective lenses in their glasses who had no eye symptoms but did have burns on the face. Eleven of the eighteen affected people sought medical care.

Of the eighteen affected patients, seventeen were seated at or standing near the back of the gymnasium. The authorities then contacted all thirty persons sitting in this high-risk area. The attack rate for eye symptoms in this high-risk area was 46 percent.

The pattern of facial burns suggested the UV light was coming from the left. This led to the discovery of a single damaged halide lamp high in the ceiling of the gymnasium.

Metal halide lamps have an arc lighting mechanism that generates intense ultraviolet radiation along with visible light. The glass encasement filters out the ultraviolet, allowing only visible light to escape. When the glass encasement is broken or damaged, ultraviolet radiation is emitted in levels that are known to produce eye damage. This was the case in this epidemic.

The mystery of an epidemic of bad eyes in the middle of the night was solved by careful study using the case study methods of detection.

Authorities of the Tennessee State Department of Health and the Epidemic Intelligence Service (EIS) of the Centers for Disease Control were notified of the cluster of cases of photokeratitis. Faculty members of the Department of Preventive Medicine from Vanderbilt School of Medicine were called in as consultants. Their findings were reported in a 2004 *article in the Archives of Pediatric Adolescent Medicine, titled "Photokeratitis"* (volume 158: pp. 372–376). In addition to this cluster of photokeratitis, the paper reports two other clusters of patients, all caused by damaged metal halide lights in gymnasiums.

Chapter Eighteen

A Near Death from Hexing

In the spring of 1938, Dr. Drayton Doherty admitted a sixty-year-old black man to the hospital. At that time, the small hospital was located at the edge of town in an old house that had been converted into a fifteen-bed hospital. Six of the beds were located upstairs at the rear of the house in what previously served as a sleeping porch. The patient was admitted to that porch.

Dr. Doherty went on to tell me that the patient, Vance Vanders, had been ill for many weeks and had lost over fifty pounds. He looked extremely wasted and near death. His eyes were sunken and resigned to death. The clinical suspicions in those days for anyone with a wasting disease were either tuberculosis or widespread cancer. Repeated tests and chest x-rays for both of these diseases were negative, as was the physical examination. Despite a nasogastric feeding tube, Vanders continued on a downhill course, refusing to eat and vomiting whatever was put down the tube. He said repeatedly he was going to die, and he soon reached a stage of near stupor. Coming in and out of consciousness, he was barely strong enough to talk. Only then did his wife, who had stayed by his bedside, ask to talk to Dr. Doherty privately. Dr. Doherty knew both the man and the wife personally. Both worked on the farm of an acquaintance of Dr. Doherty. (This farmer, when I interviewed him later, verified the story of Vanders to me.)

The sick man's wife appeared extremely nervous and anxious. She made Dr. Doherty take a vow of complete secrecy and made him swear never to tell anyone the story she was about to tell. Here was what the wife told Dr. Doherty:

About four months before Vanders was admitted to the hospital, he'd had a "run-in" with the local witch doctor, or "voodoo priest," as he was called. It was well known that many blacks in the area practiced voodoo and that there were several priests in the area. Late one night a priest had summoned Vanders to the cemetery. The wife had not been able to uncover why Vanders was called, but only that an argument occurred. While they were arguing, the priest held a bottle of some foul-smelling liquid and waved it about Vanders's face. The priest told Vanders that he had "voodoo'd" him, saying that Vanders would die in the very near future, that there was no way out, and that even medical doctors could not save him. Vanders was doomed to die. He staggered home that evening and did not eat again. Several weeks later, he was admitted to the small hospital in a moribund state.

Neither the wife nor Vanders had come forward to tell the story because the voodoo priest had told them he would voodoo all their children and as many other people as it took to keep them silent. Terrified, especially since they had seen Vanders's illness unfold as predicted, they kept the story to themselves. Seeing that Vanders was near death, the wife came forward to tell Dr. Doherty, in hopes that he could somehow miraculously save her husband.

Dr. Doherty said he was puzzled but fascinated by the story. Knowing that Vanders was near death, he spent a lot of time that night thinking about what approach he should take. Whatever he did, he knew it had to be done right away or else Vanders would certainly die.

The next morning, with his plan in mind, Dr. Doherty came to Vanders's bedside. He had asked for all the kin to be present. Ten or more of them gathered in the six-bed ward. They were trembling and frightened to be associated with this doomed man. They pulled away from the bed as Dr. Doherty approached.

Dr. Doherty said that he announced in his most authoritative voice that he now knew exactly what was wrong with Vanders. He told them of a harrowing encounter at midnight the night before in the local cemetery, where he had lured the voodoo priest on some false pretense. Dr. Doherty said he told the priest that he had uncovered his secret voodoo and found out precisely how he had voodoo'd Vanders. At first, he said, the priest had laughed at him. Dr. Doherty said he choked the priest nearly to death against a tree until the priest described exactly what he had done to Vanders.

Here is what Dr. Doherty told Vanders and the small crowd of kin who had gathered around the bed. (They hung on every word he uttered.)

"That voodoo priest rubbed some lizard eggs into your skin, and they climbed down into your real stomach and hatched out some small lizards. All but one of them died, leaving one large one, which is eating up all your food and the lining of your body. I will now get that lizard out of your system and cure you of this horrible curse."

With that he summoned the nurse. She had, on prearrangement, filled a large syringe with apomorphine (a powerful emetic, to induce vomiting). With great ceremony, Dr. Doherty pointed the syringe to the ceiling and inspected it most carefully for several moments. He squirted the smallest amount of clear liquid into the air and lunged toward Vanders. The patient had by now gathered enough strength to be sitting up wide eyed in the bed. He pressed himself against the headboard, trying to withdraw from the injection. With dramatic motions, Dr. Doherty pushed the needle into the arm of Vanders and injected the full dose of apomorphine. With that he wheeled about, said nothing, and dramatically left the ward.

In a few minutes the nurse reported that Vanders had begun to vomit. When Dr. Doherty arrived at the bedside, Vanders was retching, one wave of spasms after another. His head was buried in a metal basin that sat on the bed. After several minutes of continued vomiting, and at a point judged to be near its end, Dr. Doherty pulled from his black bag, artfully and secretly, a green lizard. At the height of the next wave of retching he slid the lizard into the basin. He called out in a loud voice, "Look, Vance, look what has come out of you. You are now cured. The voodoo curse is lifted!"

There was an audible murmur across the room. Several relatives fell on the floor and began to moan. According to Dr. Doherty and the nurse who witnessed the event, Vanders saw the lizard through his squinted eyes, did a double take, and then jumped back to the head of the bed, eyes wide, slack jawed. He looked dazed. He did not vomit again but drifted into a deep sleep within a minute or two, saying nothing. His pulse rate was extremely slow (the exact count was not recalled), and his breathing became slow and extremely deep. This sleep/coma lasted over twelve hours and into the next morning. When he woke, Vanders was ravenous for food. He gulped down large quantities of milk, bread, some meat, and eggs before he was made to stop for fear he would rupture his stomach.

Within a week Vanders was discharged from the hospital. Within a few weeks he had regained his weight and strength. He lived another ten years or so, dying of what sounds like a heart attack, having no further encounter with the voodoo priest. No one else in the family was affected.

I knew the nurse who had witnessed the events. She confirmed Dr. Doherty's story. My uncle, Dr. Sam Kirkpatrick, Sr., a local physician, also confirmed the story, as did the farmer on whose land Vanders worked.

I did not know what to make of this strange and fascinating story. It was my first encounter with hexing and voodoo. Initially, I dismissed the story as a superstitious display of primitive ignorance. However it was evident that Vanders believed at the deepest level that he was cursed and doomed to die. I wondered how words could be so powerful that they could induce death. Can just words, mere words, have that power? It was a completely new concept to me. That was why I kept asking others to verify the story, which they did. Eventually I had to accept the story as true. I could not find a hole or crack in it.

Dr. Doherty had reversed what was almost certain to be a fatal outcome. He had done it with actions and words. He had made up a story that was plausible in the extraordinarily strange voodoo world of Vanders. Dr. Doherty was able to enter that world completely. His words and actions convinced Vanders that he was healed. Once convinced, Vanders became well.

There is no deeper mystery than the power of words—whether the words cause illness, healing, or sometimes even death.

Epilogue

Clinical medicine has many similarities to careful detective work.

Medical detective work requires going beyond the usual or obvious diagnostic jargon and terminology. The point in medical care is not simply labeling the illness with a named diagnosis; the medical detective is seeking the root cause of the patient's complaints. There are only a limited number of possible medical diagnoses, but there are an almost infinite number of possible causes for illnesses and symptoms. Consider the cat in chapter 2 with toxic rose dust sleeping on the pillow of the coalminer's wife. Or the pregnant woman in chapter 6 paralyzed by eating potassium binding clay, revealed by an old aunt. Or the young man in chapter 10 whose girlfriend pumped contaminated air under his skin. These cases fail to fall under a named medical diagnosis.

Of the nineteen cases presented here, only six arrived at a named disease diagnosis. Thirteen cases were explained only by careful listening, observations, and/or epidemiological surveys.

The true detective interviews family members, seeking their observations. He inquires about pets, travels, work habits, personal beliefs, and so on. What in the life of the patient is causing the illness? Above all, the medical detective must listen carefully to the patient repeatedly. He does this until the patient becomes his or her own detective, making observations and correlations about the circumstances and surroundings of life. The detective is searching for observations about the lived life of the patient; whether it is proximity to toxic substances, involvement with stressful personal or business relationships, or dysfunctional personal beliefs.

The medical detective knows that personal beliefs, however irrational, determine physiological responses, even attempted suicide from a placebo as in chapter 3, a near death from voodoo hexing as in chapter 18, or the mass hysteria from believed toxic fumes in the school rooms of chapter 7.

The medical detective urges the patient, especially one with chronic complaints, to reflect on two general and unspecified questions. Both unspecified questions are intended to direct the patient on an extensive mental search for causes- physical, emotional, or spiritual:

1. What are you doing in your life that you should *stop* doing?
2. What are you not doing in your life that you should *start* doing?

In this age of high technology, most of which is visual, listening to the patient becomes even more important. Consider the visual nature of most tests—CAT scans, arteriograms, ultrasound pictures, brain scans, and a myriad of visualized endoscopies. None of these require listening or hearing the patient. I sometimes wonder if our entire auditory process with patients is shutting down. We seem to be saying, "If the disease cannot be 'seen', then it does not exist". But there are illnesses that can only be heard as illustrated by some of the cases reported here.

The detective stories of this book illustrate the extreme value and need for careful listening and for engaging the patient and families in their own detective process. There is not a medical diagnosis for every set of symptoms, but there is a demonstrable cause.

True Medical Detective Stories:

Chapter Notes

Chapter One: Dr. Jim's Breasts
C. V. DiRaimondo, A. Roach, C. K. Meador, "Gynecomastia, from Exposure of Vaginal Estrogen Cream," Letter to, *New England Journal of Medicine* 1980; 302:1089–90.
Published in part in C. K. Meador, *Symptoms of Unknown Origin: A Medical Odyssey* (Nashville, TN: Vanderbilt University Press, 2005).

Chapter Two: A Young Doctor and a Coal Miner's Wife
Dr. William Hueston shared this medical mystery with me and allowed me to use his name in the story. Dr. Hueston is chairman of the Department of Family Medicine at the Medical University of South Carolina in Charleston, South Carolina.

Chapter Three: A Paradoxical Suicide Attempt
R. R. Reeves, M. E. Ladner, R. H. Hart, and R. S. Burke, "Nocebo effects with antidepressant clinical drug trial placebos." *General Hospital Psychiatry* 2007; 29:275–277.

Chapter Four: A Curious Epidemic
S. M. Standaert, J. E. Dawson, W. Schaffner, J. E. Childs, K. L. Biggie, J. Singleton, R. R. Gerhardt, M. L. Knight, and R. H. Hutcheson, "Ehrlichiosis in a Golf-Oriented Retirement Community," *New England Journal of Medicine* 1995; 333:420–5.
This story was shared with me by Dr. William Schaffner of Vanderbilt School of Medicine.

Chapter Five: A Strange Coincidence
E. Cardi, "Hiccups Associated with Hair in the External Auditory Canal—Successful Treatment by Manipulation," *New England Journal of Medicine* 1961; 263:286.

M. S. Wagner and J. S. Stapcznski, "Persistent Hiccups," *Annals of Emergency Medicine* 1982; 11:1.

Chapter Six: A Paralysis of Pregnancy
Previously published in part in C. K. Meador, *Puzzling Symptoms* (Brule:Cable Publishing, 2008).

Chapter Seven: A Mysterious Epidemic in a School
F. Sirois, "Epidemic hysteria: school outbreaks 1973–1993," *Medical Principles and Practice* 1999; 8:12–25.

T. E. Jones, A. S. Craig, D. Hoy, E. W. Gunter, D. L. Ashley, D. B. Barr, J. W. Brock, and W. Schaffner, "Mass psychogenic illness attributed to toxic exposure at a high school," *New England Journal of Medicine* 2000; 342:96–100.

C. K. Meador, "Texas Heat," *Symptoms of Unknown Origin: A Medical Odyssey* (Nashville, TN: Vanderbilt University Press, 2005).

N. M. Hadler, "If you have to prove you are ill, you can't get well: the object lesson of fibromyalgia," *Spine* 1996; 21:2397–400.

S. Wessely, "Responding to mass psychogenic illness," *New England Journal of Medicine* 2000; 342:129–30.

This story was shared with me by Dr. William Schaffner of Vanderbilt School of Medicine.

Chapter Eight: Two Cases of Pneumonia: Two Different Causes
Previously reported in part in C. K. Meador, *Symptoms of Unknown Origin: A Medical Odyssey* (Nashville, TN: Vanderbilt University Press, 2005) and C. K. Meador, *Puzzling Symptoms* (Brule:Cable Publishing, 2008).

These cases were shared with me by Dr. Allen Kaiser of Vanderbilt School of Medicine.

Chapter Nine: Under the Bridges of the Cumberland River
Personal observations, C. K. Meador.

Chapter Ten: Some Things Just Get Under Your Skin
Previously published in part in C. K. Meador, *Twentieth Century Men in Medicine* (iUniverse, Inc., 2007); C. K. Meador, *Med School* (Nasnville:Hillsboro Press, 2003); and C. K. Meador, *Puzzling Symptoms* (Brule:Cable Publishing, 2008).

Chapter Eleven: The Mystery Is Not *What*, But *Why*
Veronica's story was told in abbreviated form first in C. K. Meador, *Symptoms of Unknown Origin: A Medical Odyssey* (Nashville, TN: Vanderbilt University Press, 2005) and C. K. Meador, *Puzzling Symptoms* (Brule:Cable Publishing, 2008).

Chapter Twelve: Some Diseases Are Like Serial Killers
M. G. Koenig, A. Spickard, M. A. Cardella, and D. E. Rogers, "Clinical and Laboratory Observations on Type E Botulism in Man," *Medicine* 1964; 43:517–45.
These stories were shared with me by Dr. Anderson Spickard, Jr., of Vanderbilt School of Medicine.

Chapter Thirteen: Some People Just Make You Sick
Published in part in C. K. Meador, *Symptoms of Unknown Origin: A Medical Odyssey* (Nashville, TN: Vanderbilt University Press, 2005).

Chapter Fourteen: The Case of Mrs. Oliver Townwell
A brief account was published in C. K. Meador, *Puzzling Symptoms* (Brule:Cable Publishing, 2008).

Chapter Fifteen: Pigs and Pacifiers
T. F. Jones, S. C. Buckingham, C. A. Bopp, E. Ribot, and W. Schaffner, "From Pig to Pacifier: Chitterling-Associated Yersiniosis Outbreak Among Black Infants," *Emerging Infectious Diseases* 2003; 9:1007–9.
This case was shared with me by Dr. William Schaffner of Vanderbilt School of Medicine.

Chapter Sixteen: The Nurse Solves the Mystery
Previously published in part in C. K. Meador, *Puzzling Symptoms* (Brule:Cable Publishing, 2008).

Chapter Seventeen: An Outbreak of Bad Eyes

D. L. Kirschle, T. F. Jones, N. M. Smith, and W. Schaffner, "Photokeratitis and UV-Radiation Associated with Damaged Metal Halide Lamps," *Archive of Pediatrics and Adolescent Medicine* 2004; 158:372–6.
This story was shared with me by Dr. William Schaffner of Vanderbilt School of Medicine.

Chapter Eighteen: A Near Death from Hexing

C.K. Meador, "All Some Patients Need Is Listening and Talking," *Symptoms of Unknown Origin: A Medical Odyssey* (Nashville, TN: Vanderbilt University Press, 2005).
C. K. Meador, "Hex Death: VooDoo Magic or Persuasion," *Southern Medical Journal* 1992; 85:244–47.
This story was told on the Discovery Health BBC TV channel in 2003 and later on Australian Television in 2011.

About the Author

Dr. Clifton K. Meador, born in Alabama in 1931, attended Vanderbilt School of Medicine in Nashville, where he graduated with top honors. He completed his internship and began his residency at Columbia Presbyterian Hospital in New York, then spent two years in the Army Medical Corps before completing his residency and National Institutes of Health Fellowship in Endocrinology at Vanderbilt.

During his long and varied medical career, Dr. Meador directed the NIH Clinical Research Center in Alabama, served as dean of the School of Medicine at the University of Alabama in Birmingham, created the Vanderbilt teaching service at Saint Thomas Hospital in Nashville, Tennessee, and trained young doctors as professor of medicine at Vanderbilt University and Meharry Medical College. For the past ten years, he has served as executive director of the Meharry Vanderbilt Alliance, a foundation that supports a collaborative clinical, educational, research, and training program for Meharry Medical College and Vanderbilt University.

Dr. Meador has published extensively in the medical literature; he is perhaps best known for "The Art and Science of Nondisease" and "The Last Well Person," both published in the *New England Journal of Medicine*; "A Lament for Invalids," published in the *Journal of the American Medical Association*; and "*Clinical Man: Homo Clinicus*", published in *Pharos*. The articles are satiric treatments of the excesses of medical practice.

Dr. Meador is the author of many popular medical books, including *Symptoms of Unknown Origin, Puzzling Symptoms, Little Book of Doctors' Rules, Little Book of Nurses' Rules,* and *Med School.* He enjoys woodworking, golf (a goal is to shoot his age), and his favorite hobby—writing. Meador is the proud father of seven children. He is married to Ann Cowden, an accomplished portrait artist.

Made in the USA
Las Vegas, NV
24 February 2024

86245309R00056